ETHICAL ISSUES IN REPRODUCTIVE MEDICINE

Also by Maurice Reidy

FOUNDATIONS FOR A MEDICAL ETHIC

ETHICAL ISSUES IN REPRODUCTIVE MEDICINE

Edited by Maurice Reidy

GILL AND MACMILLAN

First published by
Gill and Macmillan Ltd
Goldenbridge
Dublin 8
with associated companies in
London, New York, Delhi, Hong Kong,
Johannesburg, Lagos, Melbourne,
Singapore, Tokyo

7171 1261 6

Origination by Healyset, Dublin
Printed in Great Britain by Biddles Ltd, Guildford and Kings Lynn

Contents

Introduction 1
Maurice Reidy
1. Prenatal Diagnosis: Situating the Ethical Questions 4
Dermot MacDonald
2. Genetic Counselling 12
Joseph Masterson
3. Abortion 21
John Murphy
4. Psychological Aspects of Termination of Pregnancy 32
Noel Walsh
5. The Treatment of Infertility: Ethical Issues 45
Niall Duignan
6. Natural Family Planning 53
John Bonnar
7. Natural Family Planning: Personal Aspects 74
Dorothy Scally
8. Medico-moral Problems in the Management of Congenital Malformation 87
Edward Guiney
9. Ethical Issues in Reproductive Medicine: A Legal Perspective 95
William Binchy
10. Ethical Issues in Reproductive Medicine: from the Perspective of Moral Theology 118
Maurice Reidy

APPENDICES

1. A Note on the Nursing Care of Congenitally Malformed Infants 149
Josephine Mulligan
2. Sacred Congregation for the Doctrine of the Faith: Declaration on Euthanasia 151
3. Archdiocese of Dublin: Ethical Code for Hospitals 158
4. Ethical Principles of the Coombe Lying-In Hospital, Dublin 162
5. Excerpt from the Ethics Code of the Irish Medical Council (Comhairle na nDochtuiri Leighis) 165

Notes 166

Contributors

William Binchy, B.A., B.C.L., LL.M., Barrister-at-law, Research Counsellor, Law Reform Commission, Dublin

John Bonnar, M.A., M.D., F.R.C.O.G., Professor of Obstetrics and Gynaecology, University of Dublin, Trinity College Unit, Rotunda Hospital, Dublin

Niall M. Duignan, M.D., M.A.O., M.R.C.O.G., Master, Coombe Lying-In Hospital, Dublin

Edward Guiney, M.D., M.Ch., F.R.C.S., F.R.C.S.I., Consultant Pediatric Surgeon, Our Lady's Hospital, Director, Children's Research Centre, Our Lady's Hospital for Sick Children, Crumlin, Dublin, Professor of Pediatric Research, University College, Dublin.

Dermot MacDonald, M.B., M.A.O., F.R.C.P.I., F.R.C.O.G., Master, National Maternity Hospital, Dublin

Joseph Masterson, M.D., B.Ch., B.A.O., M.Sc., F.R.C.P.I., F.R.C.Path., Professor of Medical Genetics, University College, Dublin

Josephine Mulligan, S.R.S.C.N., S.R.N., S.C.M., Research Assistant, Children's Research Centre, Our Lady's Hospital for Sick Children, Crumlin, Dublin

John F. Murphy, M.D., F.R.C.P.I., M.R.C.O.G., Consultant Obstetrician and Gynaecologist, National Maternity Hospital, Dublin

Maurice Reidy, D.D., Faculty of Theology, Holy Cross College, Clonliffe, Dublin

Dorothy Scally, Counsellor and Tutor in Natural Family Planning Methods, Dublin

Noel Walsh, F.R.C.P.I., F.R.C.P.C., F.R.C.Psych., Professor of Clinical Psychiatry, University College, Dublin and St Vincent's Hospital, Elm Park, Dublin

Introduction

An incoming tide moves along the empty strand, front edges creeping, seeking, inching forward. This image suggests itself to my mind when I think of the way in which life reproduces itself. Viewed from a certain angle, the human race appears as a brimming source of energy, constantly pressing forward, constantly renewing itself from within. The leading edges are every mother and father and baby.

At the present time, advanced technology and rapid social change have caught up with these leading edges. Science has given us a new perception of beautiful things: the tiny unfolding of a human being, the deep familial processes of men and women. The spirit of the times has given us a renewed appreciation of human sexuality: a gift that is joyful, and not only dutiful.

Unlike the incoming tide, however, human life grows only at the edges; the idea of an unfathomable ocean of life lying behind the individual couple is an illusion. What lies behind is in the past, in the psycho-social and genetic influences from which the present moment issues forth. The new person comes from within the couple, and the first food is the nourishment and the affection which the human couple provide from their own store. The couple is supported and encouraged, or ought to be, by the wider community.

Unfortunately the picture is not all positive. There has taken place an erosion of the traditional values which urged respect for life. The accepted ethical bearings of previous generations of doctors, nurses and parents are being challenged throughout society. For many people the shoreline has begun to take on the appearance of an ethical wilderness.

The origin of this book was a series of study evenings held at the Coombe Lying-in Hospital, Dublin. The idea was to 'think through' some of the main developments in reproductive medicine. The participating group consisted of consultants to the different maternity hospitals in the city, midwife tutors and clergy who are engaged in the teaching of Medical Ethics to student nurses.

The general approach tended to be factual and analytical. It was felt that the purpose of the exercise would be best served by excluding polemic. The emphasis, therefore, rested on an up-to-date presentation of accurate knowledge, to be accompanied by considered ethical comment. It will be seen that some of the chapters concentrate on a careful presentation of facts, others offer a blend of fact and value-judgment coming from the experience and conviction of the individual author, while others address themselves to values and ethics as the principle theme.

Each chapter originated in a paper read first to the study group, where the issues involved were discussed with the author. In most cases this discussion has contributed greatly to the final form in which the paper has been published. As far as possible, the language has been kept accessible to the non-medical reader.

There is a definite editorial perspective. As a moral theologian I have sought to bring together a coalescence of evidence and opinion which will help to inform and enlighten the judgments of conscience in issues of reproductive medicine. Naturally in some areas conclusions have been more tentative, more open-ended, than in others. This is the nature of ethics, as indeed of any science.

The book begins at the pre-birth stage. Prenatal diagnosis and genetic counselling are at the forefront of advanced technology, and of ethical decision-making. Dr MacDonald, who writes on prenatal diagnosis, is widely experienced in gynaecology and obstetrics, and his professional writings include work on infertility, labour and family planning. Professor Masterson has formally initiated genetic counselling services in the Republic of Ireland in the last ten years, and in addition to his academic appointment he is consultant in Clinical Genetics to two of Dublin's major hospitals, the Mater and Our Lady's Hospital for Sick Children.

The next two chapters concentrate on the problem of abortion. Dr Murphy looks at the vital question of ethical argumentation and insists on the importance of the reasoned approach. He has been associated with 'pro-life' movements in England and in Ireland for several years, and he is well known in the medical world for his research on cervical cancer. Professor Walsh, whose academic and clinical background embraces Ireland and Canada, takes up the vital practical question as to how the woman who has had an abortion can be helped when she seeks to make good that which has been lost.

The next three chapters are concerned with fertility; the first with treatment of infertility, and the other two with fertility management. Dr Duignan's work in the field of infertility is known at national and international levels, especially his research on problems relating to ovulation. Professor Bonnar, who gives a thorough exposition of the scientific basis of natural family planning, is a consultant to the World Health Organisation special programme for Research and Training in Human Reproduction, and was Principal Investigator (for Ireland) of the WHO Multi-Centre Study of the Ovulation Method (1979). Mrs Scally is a tutor and counsellor in Natural Family Planning, and in her chapter she gives us the benefit of her experience as one who has helped many couples in different circumstances with this important, intimate and frequently anxious aspect of their lives. She is a member of the Board of the Coombe Hospital.

The book then moves into an area that is beginning to dominate the ethical headlines in the eighties, the treatment of severely handicapped babies. Professor Guiney will be familiar to many readers on account of his contribution to pediatric medicine and research, and for his writing on the treatment of infants with spina bifida. The ethical problems in this area are taken up at some length in my own chapter, and the book's handling of this difficult issue is complemented by two items in the appendix, a Note on the Nursing Care of Infants with Congenital Malformations not amenable to Surgical Intervention, by Josephine Mulligan, and the Declaration on Euthanasia, issued by the Holy See in 1980. These may be seen as a whole package in which the practical and theoretical issues are presented side by side.

The sequence of chapters concludes with the legal and the moral themes. Mr Binchy has written much on medico-legal subjects and is joint author, with Professor Bryan McMahon, of *Irish Law of Torts*. His chapter is a remarkable overview, on a world scale, of the legal doctrines that have accompanied the scientific and ethical developments which medicine has embarked upon in recent years. My own contribution attempts to review the themes of the book in the light of moral theology. It was my association with the teaching of Medical Ethics in Dublin's training hospitals, and with the people who are engaged in this work, which created the opportunity of organising this project on ethics and reproductive medicine.

There are three other items of particular interest to be found in the Appendix. One is an excerpt from the *Guide to Ethical Conduct* published in 1981 by The Medical Council (Comhairle na nDochtuiri Leighis). This excerpt is headed 'Reproductive Medicine' and it is an important statement of principle by the medical profession in Ireland. The second item is the Ethical Code for Hospitals of the Archdiocese of Dublin, which came into use in December 1978. The third is 'Principles of General Policy' as set out by the Board of the Coombe Lying-In Hospital, 1980.

I wish to record here my gratitude to the authors of the papers, who gave generously of their time and expertise. I want to thank too the participants in the discussions, and I would like to mention especially Dr John Drumm and Dr Alphonsus Greene, of the Coombe Hospital, whose interest and support contributed much to the success of the venture, and subsequently, to the clarification of certain aspects of my own paper. Finally, I thank Dr Niall Duignan, Master of the Coombe, for his assistance throughout.

Reverend Maurice Reidy

1

Prenatal Diagnosis: Situating the Ethical Questions

DERMOT MacDONALD

The term prenatal diagnosis refers to the diagnosis or detection of certain normal or abnormal conditions in the embryo, foetus or baby prior to birth.

For many years it has been possible to detect some abnormalities in the unborn baby, either by clinical signs, or more accurately by X-ray. These methods, however, were only useful when the pregnancy was well advanced, perhaps from twenty weeks at the very earliest. Today it is possible to detect some abnormalities with great accuracy at a much earlier stage of pregnancy. Among the more notable of these abnormalities are spina bifida or neural tube defect, and Down's syndrome. The method that is used is amniocentesis.

Amniocentesis

Amniocentesis is the examination of a specimen of *liquor amnii* – that is the water surrounding the baby. The estimation of the bilirubin content of this was the first breakthrough in prenatal diagnosis, and this in turn led to the first direct attempts to treat a baby *in utero*, that is, treatment of a baby before birth.

Many babies, in cases of severe jaundice and anaemia, as a result of blood group incompatibility, were saved by a transfusion of fresh adult blood given directly into their bodies while still *in utero*.

This form of treatment continues to reduce mortality in cases of severe haemolytic disease due to rhesus immunisation. Fortunately, the successful prevention of haemolytic disease in recent years has resulted in a diminishing place for this particular form of intra-uterine or prenatal diagnosis and treatment.

The most recent series of developments, however, result from the discovery that babies with neural tube defects produce a high level of a substance known as alpha feta protein (AFP). This is an amino acid.

The neural tube is a closed tubular system by the thirtieth day of pregnancy. This tube is the embryonic forerunner of the central nervous system. But failure to close may result in various forms of spina bifida or of anencephaly. The overall incidence of this kind of condition appears to be between 1 and 2 per 1,000; in Ireland, however, it is currently 4 per 1,000.

Where there is neural tube defect, AFP is found in high quantities in the mother's circulation. It is also found in high quantities in the *liquor amnii*. So if AFP is detected in large amounts in the mother's circulation during the second trimester of pregnancy, specifically between week 16 and 20, this indicates a high risk of neural tube defect. This possibility can be clarified by an examination of AFP levels in the *liquor amnii.*

It must be stressed, however, that both the plasma and the *liquor amnii* estimations of AFP must be performed between 16 and 20 weeks for accurate and reliable results. It must also be noted that some other conditions, such as twins, or foetal heart abnormalities, may also result in high levels of plasma and liquor AFP. This can also be true where the foetus is dead or where there has been wrong gestation.

Another development in the field of prenatal diagnosis is the discovery of the sex of the baby. This information can be derived from an examination of cells from the baby's skin. These cells can be collected from a specimen of liquor and the presence or absence of peripheral nuclei – called Barr bodies – indicate whether the foetus is male or female. Barr bodies in the majority of cells suggest a female foetus. The sex of the unborn baby can be determined more accurately by culturing the cells taken from the *liquor amnii* and determining their chromosome content.

A most significant development resulted from the discovery in 1959 by Lejeune that children with Down's syndrome, or mongolism, had an additional 21st chromosome – referred to as trisomy 21. This meant that certain abnormalities associated with abnormal chromosome patterns could be detected. Mongolism was the first and most important of these conditions.

Other conditions which can be diagnosed prenatally by culture and examination of the skin cells of the foetus include all autosomal trisomies and X chromosomal polysomes, such as 47XXY and 47XXX, which are very rare. The culture of these cells is a highly sophisticated laboratory procedure taking up to six weeks. The cells may occasionally fail to grow or may give a false reading as a result of chromosomal aberrations *in vitro.*

Amniocentesis therefore has become the accepted technique for prenatal diagnosis of open neural tube defects, mongolism and other chromosomal abnormalities, as well as for detecting the sex of the child.

The technique involves the passage of a needle, under local anaesthesia through the anterior abdominal wall and the uterine wall of the mother into the amniotic sac. The availability of ultrasound to determine the exact location of the placenta has made the procedure more safe. Ultrasound is also helpful in confirming the gestation of the foetus, thus ensuring that it is between 16 and 20 weeks. In addition, of course, the possibility of twins must be excluded, and it must be confirmed that the foetus is alive. Ultrasound thus minimises the possibility of misreading high AFP levels. Furthermore the localisation of the placenta will ensure that the needle does not go through this spongy organ before reaching a pool of *liquor amnii*.

Nevertheless, amniocentesis has intrinsic risks including subsequent abortion,[1] infection in the uterus, disturbance of the placenta or even direct injury to the baby by the point of the needle,[2] blood group sensitisation and, finally, amniotic fluid infusion. The overall complication rate from amniocentesis is about 2 per cent. The overall foetal loss rate in pregnant mothers who undergo amniocentesis is reported as 3.5 per cent compared to 3.2 per cent in a control group – not a statistical difference.[3] However, a British collaborate study showed a significantly higher foetal loss rate among the study group, 2.6 per cent compared to 1.1 per cent among the control group.[4]

Attempts at amniocentesis are successful in about 98 per cent of cases. Failure may relate to insufficient volume of liquor, uterine abnormality or obesity. An estimated 50,000 amniocenteses have been performed throughout the world with only one maternal death reported – due to sepsis. The risks are minimised by an experienced careful operator carrying out the procedure and succeeding first time in obtaining the required specimen of liquor.

In addition to examining the liquor for AFP content and examining the foetal cells for chromosomal abnormalities, the liquor can also be examined for certain biochemical defects such as galactosaemia or congenital adrenal hyperplasia or other inborn errors of metabolism such as Tay Sach's disease. There is a list of about 50 such conditions – most of which are due to enzymatic defects – all of which are extraordinarily rare but can be diagnosed prenatally.

Foetoscopy

A further advance in prenatal diagnosis is referred to as foetoscopy in which the foetus is actually inspected *in utero* with the aid of a fibre optic channel. This channel can be passed into the amniotic sac through a needle rather similar to but larger than that used for amniocentesis. The foetus can be inspected and even a specimen of its skin or of its blood from one of the vessels in the placenta can be taken by a fine needle sited in a vessel under direct vision. This has little practical application but is used to diagnose rare blood conditions such as sickle cell anaemia or Beta thalassaemia and other hyaemoglobinopathies. These conditions are particularly common in Greek and Cypriot populations where in closed communities one in four of all children may have thalassaemia – a blood disease – at present incurable.

The procedure of foetoscopy is hazardous for the foetus, with a high risk of abortion or miscarriage of about five per cent, and with the exception of a few centres in the UK and the USA it is rarely – if ever – used.

Neural tube defect (NTD) can be diagnosed by ultrasound alone, without recourse to AFP estimation. In experienced hands all major degrees of NTD can be detected. As equipment improves the diagnosis will become even more freely available.

Risks and Probabilities

What are the risks to the mother or foetus of these procedures? In medicine, as in life in general, all advances have a price. Ultrasound has no known risks to mother or foetus. (This is in contrast with X-ray which has serious hazards.) The taking of a sample of the mother's blood for AFP has no real risks if carried out under normal precautions. Amniocentesis has serious risks already referred to. Foetoscopy is such a risk to the foetus as to be almost unacceptable except in extremely rare conditions and these should be referred to a centre specialising in the technique. The spontaneous abortion rate following the procedure is five per cent.

What are the consequences of these investigations? A mother or father may learn at 10–20 weeks gestation that their unborn child has a spina bifida or is anencephalic or has some other defect in its spinal cord. They may thus learn that their baby is likely to be paralysed from the waist down, that it will never walk, that it will never control its bladder or its bowels, that it will live life from a wheelchair and/or that it will require many operations, that it will suffer considerable pain. On the other hand, they may learn that their baby is normal.

From culture of the cells and examination of the chromosomes they may learn at 16 weeks – rarely earlier – that their baby is mongoloid or has some other defect related to its genetic make-up.

Finally, they can learn whether their unborn child is male or female – whether they are going to have a son or daughter.

In general such tests as estimation of AFP, amniocentesis, cell culture and foetoscopy are expensive and time-consuming and can only be applied to populations of pregnant mothers in which there is a significant chance of detecting a positive result. The screening of all pregnant mothers is neither practical at a medical level nor economically possible. The tests can only be applied to groups that are at particular risk.

The overall incident of trisomy 21 is approximately one per 800 live births. By contrast, at the age of 35, the chance is one in 365; at the age of 39 the risk is one in 139 and at the age of 45 one in 32.[5] The mean age for trisomy 21 is 34, so offering ante-natal diagnosis only to women aged 35 and over would result in the detection of less than 50 per cent of cases. Other chromosomal abnormalities also increase with maternal age.

It should be mentioned that as a result of the case of Becher versus

Schwartz in a New York court in 1979,[6] it is now legally obligatory in the United States to inform mothers over the age of 35 of amniocentesis and its possibilities.

Mass screening of all pregnant mothers by measuring serum levels of AFP at 16–20 weeks would result in the diagnosis of 85 per cent of cases of anencephaly and 79 per cent of open spina bifida.[7] However, great anxiety could be caused by total screening as 95 per cent of those screened will demonstrate normal levels of AFP. About two per cent of those whose plasma levels are measured will require amniocentesis. In this two per cent undergoing amniocentesis, the incidence of NTD has been reported as approximately six per cent.

Practical Questions

The questions concerning prenatal diagnosis are serious and practical. From the doctor's viewpoint, does he wait for the mother to raise the question of prenatal diagnosis or does he introduce the topic to her as part of his commitment to her ante-natal care? Does he offer amniocentesis to her if she is particularly at risk – if only to be able to reassure her that her baby has not got an NTD or is not a mongol?

From the mother's viewpoint, can she insist on amniocentesis – even for possibly frivolous reasons such as to learn the sex of her unborn baby? Will she be able to sue the doctor who does not offer amniocentesis or who refused to perform it?

One view of amniocentesis is as follows:

> Amniocentesis for ante-natal diagnosis is now an integral part of modern obstetrics and perinatal care. The procedure has been determined to be highly accurate and safe. Because of the vital consequences of the results only physicians and laboratories experienced in these procedures should undertake the responsibility of amniocentesis and amniotic fluid analysis for intra-uterine genetic diagnosis.[8]

Another assessment states:

> Amniocentesis and culture of amniotic fluid cells is relatively safe and highly accurate – greater than 99 per cent.[9]

Should amniocentesis be offered to mothers who have had repeated spontaneous abortions – knowing that perhaps 50 per cent of these may have been due to foetal anomalies – to women who have been exposed to irradiation or to harmful drugs such as chemotherapeutic agents or to those with metabolic derangements which can predispose to chromosomal abnormalities: autoimmune thyroiditis, ante-trypsin deficiencies,[10] cases of intra-uterine growth retardation?

If the risk of spontaneous abortion is one per cent, the risk of the NTD or of other abnormalities such as mongolism must be greater than this to arguably justify the procedure. Turnbull suggests that on his figures the risk is not justified under the age of 40.

Diagnosis is an information gathering procedure. A few disorders may be treated prenatally. The benefit in general of reassurance does not *at present* outweigh the risks of the procedure and so widescale screening by amniocentesis is not justified but only selective screening is acceptable and available.

The Foreseeable Future

The methods are, at present, associated with risks to the unborn baby as well as to the mother. But it is certain that those risks and complications which at present may outweigh the benefits of a positive diagnosis in all groups except those most seriously at risk will decrease. Methods are being perfected to reduce the need for such invasions of the foetal environment: prenatal diagnosis will be possible from cells collected at the neck of the womb at the uterine cervix; these cells will reflect the state of the foetus – whether it has an NTD or not, or whether it has Down's syndrome, or whether it is a boy or a girl.

Foetal squames found in the cervical canal can be cultured, or foetal lymphocytes recoverable from material circulation can be cultured for chromosomal counting.[11] Foetal lymphocytes have already been recovered and cultured from maternal blood.[12]

The mother's blood may reveal antibodies to foetal conditions. In the very near future – perhaps within a year or two – the detection of antibodies in the maternal blood may reveal the presence of a foetus who has fibrocystic disease. There will almost be no risk to the mother or the unborn foetus in prenatal diagnostic procedures. The risk of abortion or of other complications will no longer be present.

Ethical Questions

In societies where termination of pregnancy is part of normal everyday practice, more and more requests are being received for prenatal diagnosis. People want 'quality babies' and are prepared to be selective and reject the imperfect.

Of course, the answer is to find the cause of NTD, Down's syndrome, of fibrocystic disease and then prevent their occurrence. The story of haemolytic disease serves as a happy analogy, the detection of blood groups, the recognition of the incompatibility resulting in jaundice of the newborn or hydrops fetalis, the determination to treat the newborn baby by early induction and delivery followed by mutiple exchange transfusions. Subsequently intra-uterine transfusions become possible and finally, the arrival of a safe, effective method of prevention of haemolytic disease by the administration of Anti-D to the mother. A disease is dying out which killed many babies before or after birth or left many mentally retarded because of kernicterus.

Is the same process occuring in relation to NTD? The work on potato blight, on vitamin B, all point to a possible deficiency state being the cause of NTD. Will vitamin tablets given prior to conception and in the first six weeks of pregnancy be the answer to raised plasma AFP, to amniocentesis, to requests for termination? Will spina bifida be shown to be related to vitamin deficiencies? Only time will tell, but the answer to induced abortion must include an intense scientific approach to the causes of conditions for which abortion is sought.

In the meantime there are people who care for people in society. There are people who will care for spastic children, for spina bifida children: there are parents who will welcome and love a mongoloid son or daughter. There are couples who will adopt the least attractive or the most deformed children, knowing that such children prosper and grow with love, care and affection.

In general, patient-doctor consultations are on a one-to-one basis. In the very personal field of reproductive medicine, it is very important that each patient be recognised and treated as an individual with her own particular problems. The doctor must tailor his advice, his approach to the patient's problems, knowing as much as he can about the particular patient, her background, her beliefs and convictions, her attitude to her pregnancy, to her unborn baby and to the rest of the family. The relationship between the expectant mother and the doctor supervising her pregnancy is a very particular one and it is difficult to apply generalisations. Such generalisations can only be broad guidelines for dealing with individual patients.

Parents in general have the right to all the information available about the health of their children, unborn as well as born. In general such information must be given fairly, accurately, unemotionally and truthfully.

If a mother wishes to know what the particular statistical risk for her is of having a Down's syndrome baby, the medical attendant, knowing her age and her history, should state the risk. If she wishes to know whether such a complication as spina bifida can be determined early in pregnancy, she should be told the facts about AFP, amniocentesis – the risks, the accuracy of the test and the possible outcome. A mother who will not tolerate abortion may, or may not, reject such tests, while on the other hand a mother who can accept abortion may request that such tests be carried out irrespective of the risks, side effects or complications.

The doctor, of course, just as he can exercise his right to refuse to have anything to do with abortion, would have a similar obligation not to carry out such tests if they were not medically justified in his opinion. He should be able to explain to the patient the basis of these views and, of course, not undermine the patient in any way because she may not share his convictions. She, of course, has the freedom to seek another opinion.

The basis of any consultation is truth, understanding, compassion, respect for the other person's view and an overriding respect for life. A doctor committed to the Hippocratic Oath and the preservation of human life may not wish to lead a mother into a situation where she may decide to have her pregnancy terminated. Yet he has an obligation to inform her factually, to counsel her, to tell her of his own views and to allow her to make her own decisions. She will be aware of his willingness or unwillingness to carry out her wishes. Such consultations are time-consuming and need a quiet and peaceful atmosphere. The conveyor-belt type antenatal clinic is not the best place for such individual discussions.

And so, in the matter of prenatal diagnosis at present, the tests have risks, inaccuracies, are expensive, time-consuming and can only be applied to that section of the population at greatest risk of having a positive test. The results of such tests can be a great comfort when they confirm the presence of a foetus which does not have a neural tube defect, is not a Down's syndrome or has not some other detectable anomaly. On the other hand, if such an abnormality is detected the mother may request termination of the pregnancy or may live in anxious anticipation for 20 or more weeks awaiting the arrival of her defective son or daughter. She may require great support in her decision to have her baby.

The tests in their present form should not be carried out for frivolous reasons – such as just to detect the sex of the unborn child. All forms of intervention in pregnancy have risks and these risks must be balanced against any possible good that will follow from carrying out the test.

2

Genetic Counselling

JOSEPH G. MASTERSON

Several factors in the past few decades have determined the emergence of clinical genetics as a new discipline in health care services. Advances in obstetrics, infection control and blood transfusion technology have resulted in a dramatic decline in perinatal infant mortality and morbidity. There has been no corresponding reduction in the number of babies with congenital malformations and increasing attention has therefore been focused on this problem. The public, due to better health education and greater exposure to the media, are showing a lively interest in the problems of physical and mental handicap and since average family size is now much smaller than formerly, parents wish to ensure as far as possible that the few offspring they have will all be perfect. This increasing preoccupation with congenital malformations and genetically determined illness has partly stimulated, and partly derived its impetus from, highly important scientific and technical advances in cytogenetics, molecular biology and biochemistry.

Most people are surprised to learn that 2–2.5 per cent of all infants born suffer from a physical, sensory or mental handicap which is either evident at birth or becomes manifest in the early months of the child's life. The general frequency of such occurrences does little to lessen their impact on individual families. Parental shock, grief or even shame, may be compounded by feelings of guilt, isolation and biological inferiority. The emotional stability of the marriage may be threatened. Normal family activities can be severely curtailed by the sacrifice of time and money involved in the care of the handicapped child. Fears regarding possible recurrence of the handicap in future children add to the misery and confusion experienced by the parents. In such situations the clinical geneticist is an important member of the medical and paramedical team whose responsibility it is to provide all possible help and support. The services provided by the clinical geneticist are grouped together under the general heading of genetic counselling.

Genetic counselling has been defined by Carter[1] as a service to parents and potential parents aimed at providing individuals and married couples with estimates of any special extra risks of disease, malformation or handicap in any children they may have. Such risks must be put into perspective with regard to the prognosis for any child which may be affected and also in relation to the risk applicable to a random birth in the general population. The role of genetic counselling is not, of course, confined to the mere provision of risk estimates. Parents can derive psychological benefit from a clear and simple exposition of the genetic mechanism involved in their child's handicap and from an assurance that the concept of blame can never be entertained in relation to a genetic mishap. They can also be made aware of treatments and services available to their child and helped in the matter of suitable referrals for these. Finally, they can be informed about the options available to them if they consider that the recurrence risk is unacceptably high.

The extremes of orientation in genetic counselling have been the 'instructive' approach in which the counsellor confines himself to the provision of information and the 'directive' approach in which the consultants are told, with varying degrees of subtlety and paternalism, what to do on the basis of the information provided. Kessler[2] has recently argued in favour of an intermediate style in which the directive approach is eschewed but counselling nevertheless becomes person-orientated rather than purely content-orientated. Parents should not have decisions made for them but they do require sympathetic help in coming to terms with the realities and implications of their encounter with genetic disease.

The twin foundations of successful genetic counselling are precise diagnosis and an accurate family tree. A fundamental task in relation to diagnosis is confirmation that the condition in question is in fact genetically determined. There are many environmental factors in both prenatal and post-natal life which can mimic the effects of harmful genetic influences and the identification of their role in individual cases of handicap or malformation is essential if serious counselling errors are to be avoided. Precise diagnosis of a genetically determined malady may sometimes depend largely on experience and clinical acumen but there are many instances in which special investigations are needed to establish or confirm a diagnosis. The clinical geneticist must often therefore seek the help of colleagues in radiology, biochemistry, cytogenetics or haematology to arrive at the confident diagnosis on which effective counselling is based. A carefully recorded family tree is also essential since it will suffice in many instances to indicate the mode of inheritance of a particular handicap and also to identify individuals at risk apart from the consultant.

While most requests for counselling concern parents who have already had a handicapped child, an appreciable number of couples come for advice before marriage, or, if married, before starting a family. In some instances one or other member of the pair is suffering from a condition believed to be genetically determined but most pre-marital or pre-conceptional consultations are prompted by either a worrying family history or the fact that the couple concerned are blood relatives. Some engaged couples who are not related and who have impeccable family health backgrounds request pre-marital screening for hidden genetic flaws which might adversely affect their future offspring. It is necessary in such cases to explain as gently as possible, and without unduly damping their eugenic enthusiasm, that such screening, in the absence of a specific indication, is simply not possible for both technical and economic reasons. This is not to say that pre-marital screening is never of value. The high carrier frequencies of the recessive genes for sickle-cell disease, thalassaemia and Tay-Sachs disease in certain communities fully justify premarital testing for the relevant disease to detect possible marriages between carriers.

The technical achievement of Tjio and Levan[3] in 1956 of making possible the examination of human chromosomes was an outstanding landmark in human genetics. Application of their technique in subsequent years confirmed the chromosomal basis of many conditions involving mental and physical handicap, infertility and ambiguous sexual development. In some instances, e.g. Down's syndrome, the affected individual has received one chromosome too many from one or other parent and in other cases there is a deficiency of an entire chromosome (e.g. Turner's syndrome) or part of a chromosome (e.g. Cat Cry syndrome). In many cases involving an additional chromosome advancing maternal age is an undoubted factor and a large proportion of such mishaps could be avoided if child bearing could be completed by maternal age 35 years. Following the birth of a child with an additional chromosome the recurrence risk is low, of the order of one per cent, unless advanced maternal age determines a higher risk figure.

A much higher risk for an abnormal child with excessive or deficient chromosome material may exist if one or other parent is carrier of a balanced chromosome translocation. Such carriers are themselves physically and mentally normal individuals with the right amount of chromosome material in their cells – but with some rearrangement of this material involving attachment of nearly all or part of one chromosome to another one. The majority of such individuals can have normal children but will also have a high risk of having seriously handicapped chromosomally unbalanced offspring. The magnitude of this risk varies with the type of translocation and the sex of the carrier parent but it reaches its extreme in the case of a normal parent with both members of the same chromosome pair attached to one another. The writer knows a married lady with a balanced 13/13 translocation who can never have a normal child and whose offspring will invariably show the profound handicap and unsightly stigmata of Patau's syndrome. This 100 per cent risk of an abnormal child, though fortunately a rare situation, constitutes a problem of the utmost gravity for those who are concerned about the morality of sterilisation and contraception.

Spontaneous abortion loss is apparently an important natural rejection mechanism for chromosomally unbalanced embryos. Surveys have reported high frequency of chromosomal abnormality in spontaneously aborted embryos and some have put this as high as fifty per cent. An extension of this observation indicates the relevance of chromosome analysis for couples whose reproductive history includes several spontaneous abortions. The analysis will sometimes reveal an unsuspected parental balanced translocation resulting in abnormal embryos.

Counselling for monogenic conditions is basically simple and depends on the application of appropriate Mendelian ratios. In the case of handicaps determined by abnormal autosomal dominant genes we know that some affected individuals born to apparently normal parents represent sporadic fresh mutations and that recurrence risk for subsequent siblings is minimal. Autosomal dominant genes, however, are sometimes notoriously variable in the severity of their expression. Thus, the apparently healthy parents of a child profoundly handicapped by tuberous sclerosis must pass an exhaustive clinical assessment before it can be accepted that one or other of them does not possess the harmful gene with greatly diminished expression. When an individual does possess a deleterious autosomal dominant gene the prognosis for his or her offspring, irrespective of their sex, is that on average half of them will receive the gene. For some conditions the severity of handicap in those receiving the gene will be fairly predictable; in others the degree of disability may be randomly greater or less than that of the affected parent. The autosomal dominant gene for Huntington's chorea poses a particularly distressing problem in that the mental and neurological abnormalities of this condition frequently do not manifest themselves until middle age. It is difficult to imagine a more agonising dilemma than that of the children of a forty-five year-old man or woman who has started to manifest signs of Huntington's chorea. On average half of them will eventually be similarly affected but no individual can be certain whether or not he or she has inherited the gene. The only options open to such an individual are to marry and risk perpetuating the tragedy in succeeding generations or remain celibate (or at least childless) even though the possibility exists that he or she has in fact escaped the gene.

Problems determined by autosomal recessive inheritance usually arise as the result of marriage of an unsuspecting carrier of a harmful recessive gene to a similarly unaware carrier of the same harmful gene. For each offspring of such a union there is a one-in-four chance of being homozygous (i.e. receiving the harmful gene from both parents) and thus being affected by the relevant illness or handicap. Since there are three chances out of four for a normal child at each pregnancy it follows that many carrier couples having small families may have only normal offspring and never become aware of the risk to which they were exposed. The role of premarital carrier detection in relation to autosomal recessive inheritance has been referred to above. Another counselling consideration with particular relevance to this type of inheritance is the influence of consanguineous marriage on the likelihood of having affected children. Any individual carrying an abnormal recessive gene is clearly more likely to marry a carrier of the same gene if he or she marries a blood relative instead of an unrelated spouse. It is also likely that risks are increased for polygenic disorders. The effect of consanguinity is such that in the case of a union between first cousins the risk of abnormality or death in early childhood is approximately double the general population risk.

Prominent among the illnesses determined by autosomal recessive inheritance are the inborn errors of metabolism. For many of these no effective treatment has yet been devised but there are some which, if treated early enough, can be compatible with normal development. Establishment of national neonatal screening programmes for these treatable conditions represents an important achievement in preventive medicine. The discovery that treatment following early detection of these illnesses is effective now encourages known carrier parents to undertake pregnancies which would formerly have been considered too hazardous.

X-linked inheritance is not merely a phenomenon of importance to geneticists but also enjoys wide popular interest because of the occurrence of haemophilia in several of the royal houses of Europe and the fact that handicaps determined by this mechanism almost invariably affect boys. The common and relatively harmless defect of colour blindness is transmitted in this way but there are many much more serious conditions, such as the crippling and eventually lethal Duchenne muscular dystrophy, which are also X-linked. Female carriers of such genes are in general clinically normal and refined biochemical or other tests may be required to detect their carrier status. The most common marriage involved is that of a genetically normal male to a healthy but carrier female. On average, half of the boys resulting from such a mating will be affected by the relevant illness and though all girls will be clinically normal half of them on average will be carriers like their mother. The phenomenon of fresh sporadic mutation also operates in this type of inheritance and can determine that in a particular family a female may be the first individual to possess the harmful gene and have the potential of transmitting it. Similarly in a family with a negative clinical history an affected boy may be born. Such an event poses the problem of determining whether the harmful gene has lain hidden in unaffected females for one or more generations or alternatively has arisen by a process of fresh mutation in the offspring of a genetically normal mother. To distinguish between these two situations is obviously important since in the former the recurrence risk is high and in the latter it is negligible. Unfortunately reliable tests for maternal carrier status are not available in all instances.

Apart from the chromosomal and monogenic problems outlined above there are other handicaps and malformations in which twin and family studies indicate the existence of a genetic component. In these conditions the counselling precision made possible by chromosome analysis or Mendelian ratios is lacking and recurrence risks are generally of a lower though not insignificant magnitude. It is now generally accepted that these common handicaps which include spina bifida, congenital hip dislocation, congenital heart disease and some forms of mental handicap are based on predisposing polygenic influences interplaying with often unidentified environmental determinants. Risk figures for a future child depend on the number of relatives already affected and sometimes on the severity of the lesions in the affected relative. In many of these conditions recurrence risks are of the order of 3 – 5 per cent if there is already one affected first-degree relative, and 8 – 12 per cent if there are two. For any such illness or malformation the recurrence risk figures have not been calculated on the basis of predictable ratios but have to be determined empirically by the study of many families in which children have been born subsequent to the birth of one or more handicapped individual.

There are several options available to a couple who have received a worrying prognosis for future pregnancies. The first of these is to accept the risk and proceed with a further pregnancy or pregnancies. This may be the only option in those situations where the couple desperately want a child of their own and would not countenance pre-natal diagnosis and selective abortion. In some marriages there are great resources of religious faith, courage and emotional stability which make such a course seem less daunting than it would otherwise be. On the other hand it can be a recipe for disaster when a diminished sense of responsibility is compounded by disaffection and instability in the marriage relationship.

Couples unwilling to take such risks may simply decide not to have any children of their own and, if possible, to establish a family by adoption. Such a decision raises the problem of effective long-term family planning which can be particularly difficult in the case of a young couple. It would seem that sexual abstinence, though undoubtedly effective, would involve a level of heroic restraint beyond the capabilities of most couples. So-called natural family planning based on restriction of sexual activity to the infertile period also makes demands of discipline and restraint which may be beyond the intellectual or behavioural capabilities of some husbands and wives. Even if conscientiously practised, this approach to family limitation may have the disadvantage of not guaranteeing the full effectiveness demanded by the serious implications of a possible pregnancy. The same criticism can be applied to mechanical and chemical methods of contraception. With other methods there are also problems both physical and moral, in that prolonged use of 'the pill' is known to constitute a health hazard for the mother and some forms of hormonal contraception as well as the intrauterine coil are more likely to be early abortifacients than actual contraceptives.

Faced with such difficulties a young couple might consider that surgical sterilisation of one or other partner offers the most effective and acceptable solution. In view of the frequent failure to restore fertility by reparative surgery after vasectomy or tubal ligation, a decision regarding sterilisation must never be lightly taken. The prospect of irreversibility must be clearly accepted and again the stability of the marriage should be beyond reasonable doubt before taking such a serious step. Vasectomy is, from a surgical point of view, a simpler procedure than tubal ligation but the possibility of long-term unwanted effects on the systemic vasculature has recently been suggested. Tubal ligation requires an abdominal operation which, even though it must be classified as a minor procedure, nevertheless involves the small risk involved in any surgical intervention. There is for both procedures the possibility of psychological repercussions in that, despite unimpaired sexual performance, the woman may feel less a woman and the man may feel that somehow he has sacrificed an aspect of his virility. The decision regarding which partner is to be sterilised would be dictated by the circumstances of the case. A husband whose mother had just developed Huntington's chorea would obviously be the one to undergo the procedure. The woman with the 13/13 translocation referred to above or a female carrier of a seriously incapacitating X-linked gene would be the rational choice in their respective marriages. Such decisions are based on the fact that it is always possible that the genetically involved individual may die from some unrelated cause and the surviving partner might wish to remarry and have children. In the case of autosomal recessive inheritance where both partners are carriers, the choice is an open one but may be influenced by the fact that vasectomy is a less serious procedure and will leave unimpaired the wife's possibility of having a baby by donor artificial insemination (AID).

Artificial insemination by donor sperm is urged today in a number of genetically hazardous situations. If the husband is suffering, or likely to suffer, from an autosomal dominant condition with its attendant 1 in 2 risk to offspring, if he has a balanced chromosome translocation or if he carries the same harmful autosomal recessive gene as his wife, AID offers the highest possibility of a normal child for his wife. Sperm donors are selected with care on the basis of their physical and intellectual attributes and their anonymity is scrupulously preserved. The procedure is not, however, immune to the general population risk of an offspring with some kind of handicap and the knowledge that his wife's baby is not his own biological offspring may place a heavy strain on the emotional equanimity of the husband. There are, furthermore, serious moral questions here, and legal difficulties regarding the status of the child, and these could subsequently aggravate an already difficult situation.

In recent years the aspect of clinical genetics which has been most enthusiastically developed and implemented is that of ante-natal diagnosis and selective abortion of affected foetuses. In most instances this involves taking a sample of amniotic fluid from the sac surrounding the foetus early in the second trimester of pregnancy. Foetal cells in this fluid can be subjected to diagnostic chromosome analysis and studies of disturbed cellular metabolism. The fluid itself can also be analysed for abnormal constituents. Thus anencephaly and nearly all cases of open spina bifida can be diagnosed by the raised levels of alphafetoprotein found in the fluid in these common conditions. Some tests may take three weeks or longer to complete so that if amniocentesis is performed at fifteen weeks, the couple must be prepared to accept a termination at eighteen weeks or sometimes later. In some X-linked conditions there is no reliable ante-natal diagnostic test but foetal sex is always easily determinable. Since these conditions affect only males a carrier mother may elect to have all male foetuses aborted even though half of these on average will be normal.

Accurate localisations of intrauterine structures by ultrasound has increased the safety and efficiency of amniocentesis. The procedure nevertheless involves a slightly increased risk of abortion, an increased risk of eventual postural orthopaedic abnormalities in the baby and an overall increase of almost one per cent in perinatal mortality.[4] Some skeletal abnormalities and external malformations are not susceptible to diagnosis by examination of amniotic fluid but can be identified by radiography or actual inspection of the foetus with flexible fibreoptic instruments (foetoscopy). The former procedure involves the small teratogenic and carcinogenic risks associated with diagnostic levels of radiation and the latter carriers a five to ten per cent risk of abortion even when performed by experienced operators.

There is no doubt that ante-natal diagnosis and selective abortion can reduce the number of malformed and handicapped children born by extinguishing life before birth. It can furthermore be argued that the availability of these procedures encourages many couples, who would otherwise be fearful to do so, to embark on pregnancies frequently resulting in healthy offspring. There are also cases in which the sheer hardship of the situation represents an emotionally persuasive argument in favour of such expedients. The writer, for example, knows a young and devoted couple whose entire family consists of two boys with spina bifida and one with muscular dystrophy. The inescapable fact of abortion is, however, that the life of a human foetus is extinguished. Many couples, who would find the less drastic expedients of sterilisation or AID acceptable in pressing circumstances, are adamant in refusing to consider pregnancy termination. Many physicians likewise find it unacceptable that their role in the care of a handicapped human being should be to terminate its life. Others, both couples and physicians, perceive only the immediate benefit of preventing the birth of a malformed or handicapped child. It would seem that such individuals either fail to appreciate the reality of what is involved in abortion or, if they do appreciate it, succeed in blurring that reality and suppressing any moral misgivings they may feel.

It is easy for a couple who have had only normal children, or for individuals who have never had to care for a severely handicapped child, to proclaim the immorality of so-called therapeutic abortion. Their protestations must lack conviction, however, if they remain indifferent to the plight of those who have been less lucky in the reproductive lottery. Effective genetic counselling can do much to prevent the procreation of handicapped children but only generous material and emotional help from the general population can support the courage and sacrifice of those who respect the right to life of their less than perfect children.

3

Abortion

JOHN F. MURPHY

Abortion, defined for the purposes of this chapter as the wilful termination of a pregnancy, known to have commenced, with the aim of killing the foetus, is a subject that still excites much passion.

Between the advocates of liberal abortion and those who reject it under any circumstances there is almost an unbridgeable gulf. Yet it is a subject which can deeply touch the hearts of those who think about it, whatever their belief, because it is concerned with human life and man's 'right' and ability to destroy it. For the contemporary humanist liberal, abortion represents an essential human freedom, while for the committed pro-life campaigner it represents the last line of defence, the *ne plus ultra*. Real dialogue between these two extreme groups has become almost impossible.

Abortion has, of course, been part of many societies for centuries. Physicians in ancient Rome administered all manner of 'medicines' to women inconveniently pregnant. The criminal, back street or septic abortionist has been with us for generations. So, also, has the medically qualified racketeer, willing to risk his reputation and licence for handsome rewards.

In the world at present an estimated 30–55 million abortions are performed each year, making abortion one of the most prevalent means of fertility control; so much so that in many countries, especially in the Eastern European group and Japan, easy abortion has become society's norm. In 1978, the latest year for which figures are available 1,157,776 legally advised abortions were carried out in the United States.[1] The majority (sixty per cent) of the world's population lives in countries where abortion is permitted either on request or for social reasons.

Because abortion has become almost endemic in so many parts of the world, mostly 'developed' ones, and because in most of these countries a sizeable group remains utterly opposed to it, the whole development of the clamour for easy abortion and the opposition to it are worthy of detailed examination.

In recent years the number of countries which have introduced laws permitting the termination of pregnancy, has increased and in almost all these countries there have been subsequent efforts to repeal or modify such legislation. At the beginning of any campaign to liberalise the laws concerning abortion the promoters have usually advanced their cause primarily on medical grounds. Tragic case histories of women dying because of a continuing pregnancy were cited, eliciting much public and, consequently, political sympathy. Abortion was portrayed as a 'life-saving' and therapeutic procedure. The next phase was usually the extension of the concept of health to include adverse psychological or social consequences to the mother or indeed to the whole family. Liberal abortion was depicted as a social boon, protecting women and families from the ravages of overcrowding, poor opportunities, depression, etc. The next phase was often the advocacy of abortion when a child prior to birth was known to be deformed or when it was judged that if a child was born it would be at high risk of having or transmitting some disease (e.g. haemophilia). In consequence of this, huge efforts have been put into ante-natal diagnosis with many millions of pounds expended over the past decade on efforts to diagnose certain, usually very rare, congenital disorders.

Finally, and predictably, all this has led to abortion on demand. The direction of arguments in favour of abortion have usually moved from medical to ideological and to questions of social justice and individual rights (never those of the foetus). From this has evolved a concept that will be difficult to change, that a woman has an absolute right and freedom to dispose of her individual pregnancy without reference to the wishes of the father of the child or to her other children, or to the community in general. In many countries the concept of the 'right' to dispose of a pregnancy has become a subject of increasingly permissive legislation with the direction of much legislation moving predictably from medical to ideological issues, to questions of social justice and personal rights.

It has been found important to invoke the law, for legislation, no matter how poorly conceived or badly implemented, lends a powerful respectability to any procedure, and the enormous influence and protection of secular legislation can profoundly affect the attitude of persons – individually and collectively. Nowhere has this been more obvious than in the United Kingdom where the week the Abortion Act was passed in 1967 the Registrar of the General Medical Council wrote to the British Medical Journal saying that, as it was no longer illegal to perform abortions under the terms of the Act, it (the GMC) would no longer prosecute doctors who did so. The day before the Act was passed abortion was a matter of infamous professional conduct which usually led to erasure from the Register, thus depriving a doctor of his facilities to practice. In general, legislation on abortion has included a conscience clause absolving a doctor or para-medical persons, such as nurses, with ethical objections to the procedure, from becoming involved. Nonetheless, there is frequently an 'invisible pressure' placed on doctors and others to conform with what is believed to be the dominant social attitude. The arguments used to justify abortions are usually threefold: medical, psychiatric and social. These will now be individually examined.

The Medical Argument

The pressure to introduce legislation permitting abortion or to liberalise existing legislation has usually commenced with the exhibition of individual tragic case histories annotating women who, it was alleged, could not physically cope with a continuing pregnancy. It is somewhat of a paradox that however valid these arguments might have been some generations ago, with the advances in medical treatment during the past number of decades they have almost no validity now. It is not an exaggeration to state that in the current practice of medicine in Western communities there is no incidence where a continuing pregnancy would result in the death of a mother and where interruption of that pregnancy would ensure her survival.

In an authoritative review article Rovinsky and Gusberg (1967) found that between the years 1954–1964 there was a stable incidence of 'medical indications to terminate a pregnancy' of 12 per 10,000 deliveries.[2] The common medical indications were: malignancy, cardiac disease, renal disease, pulmonary disease and gastro-intestinal disease, in that order. That would mean that in the National Maternity Hospital in Dublin there would be some ten patients 'requiring termination' each year. Study of the annual reports of the National Maternity Hospital over many years, or indeed of any maternity hospital shows that this, of course, is far from the truth.

The tragic presence of malignant disease in a pregnant woman brings forth some of the most emotive arguments in favour of pregnancy termination. When the problem is examined unemotionally it has to be stated, and stated clearly, that, in general, pregnancy and malignancies of all types develop independently of each other with little reciprocal effects. Treatment may be similarly independent in most patients. In situations of advanced malignancy where only palliation is possible abortion is pointless and indeed may be psychologically harmful. When the cancer is amenable to treatment this should be carried out without disturbance to the pregnancy and currently many protective techniques are available to reduce any hazard to the foetus from specific modalities of treatment. If, however, access to treatment is interfered with by the pregnancy, as in cases of cervical or ovarian cancer in early pregnancy, definitive treatment should be, in my opinion, carried out despite the presence of the pregnancy. The prognosis for breast cancer was, at one time, considered to be worse if a pregnancy was present and termination was advised with, for many, the raising of all the old and largely unhelpful arguments of mother versus baby. Current knowledge now indicates that the presence of a pregnancy has no effect on the natural history of breast cancer, and breast cancer or its treatment has no specific effect on pregnancy.

Similarly with heart disease. It has now been known for some time (O'Driscoll *et al.*, 1962)[3] that with good medical and surgical care and with the co-operation of the patient, abortion is never indicated for patients with heart disease. The position could be argued slightly differently for women with chronic kidney disease, as occasionally such women can develop a very acute illness in the middle months of pregnancy. These patients usually have hypertension (raised blood pressure). The course of these diseases, however, is most unpredictable and it is almost impossible to say which patient will develop a serious complication refractory to ordinary therapy. In the proceedings (Bonnar *et al*, 1980)[4] of the first meeting of the International Society of Hypertension in Pregnancy there was not a single reference to the need for termination of pregnancy, and this was in a book of over 500 pages containing more than 100 papers on aspects of the subject ranging from the highly experimental to the most practical.

In summary, it may be said that there is virtually no obvious case for abortion in order to save the mother's life or to promote good health in the mother. All this, of course, presupposes that the patient is willing to take the proffered medical advice concerning the management of her pregnancy. This can involve considerable inconvenience for the mother and her family, necessitating long periods of hospitalisation, etc. Very often the advice to terminate a pregnancy on medical grounds is loaded, understandably, with such considerations and also with the potential ability of the mother to subsequently look after her growing child. And so, it must be re-stated that a situation never arises where the continuation of a pregnancy represents a serious challenge to a mother's health and where abortion would safely remove this challenge, provided always that the mother is willing to take appropriate medical advice.

The Psychiatric Argument

With the phenomenal advances in medical and obstetric care over the past fifty years, even the most ardent abortionist would agree that from the standpoint of physical medicine the number of abortions that could be genuinely termed therapeutic is minuscule, if it exists at all. On the other hand, the 'indications' for abortion on psychiatric grounds are increasing. In the already cited study of Rovinsky and Gusberg (1967) the psychiatric indications for abortion rose from 24 to 56 per 100,000 deliveries. More and more patients in countries with liberal abortion laws are being referred to psychiatrists for a decision on the desirability of continuing a pregnancy. The opinions of psychiatrists also vary greatly from those who hold that there is no psychiatric reason for abortion to those who believe that the pressures of an inconvenient pregnancy represent an emotional risk to the patient and that the pregnancy is, therefore, best terminated.

Myre Sim, now at the University of Toronto and lately of Birmingham, England, has been an important and persistent critic of abortion on psychiatric grounds. He states that in his experience, and especially in his wide experience of dealing with patients who have had puerperal psychosis, there is no psychiatric indication for abortion.

Sim believes that the treatment of psychosis whether the patient is pregnant or not, is psychotherapy and that surgery to empty the womb has no place in this regimen. Sim further believes that with appropriate treatment even some of the most disturbed patients will not commit suicide while pregnant. In his widely acclaimed *Guide to Psychiatry* (1978) he states that in his experience post-abortive psychosis is a more resistant condition to treatment than is post-partum psychosis. For this reason any psychiatrist who recommends abortion on the basis of a previous episode of post-partum psychosis seems on very doubtful clinical ground. Similar views concerning the inadvisability of abortion on psychiatric grounds have been expressed by Karl Stern, one of Canada's outstanding psychiatrists (Walsh, 1977).[5]

In clinical practice one occasionally encounters a patient who, on learning she is pregnant, becomes depressed and may even threaten suicide. Here again the treatment is that appropriate to depression and this may, in fact, require hospitalisation. The 'hysterical threat' is well recognised: 'If you don't agree to abortion I will kill myself.' A doctor 'blackmailed' by such threats is very foolish, as to perform an abortion under such a crisis situation is often followed by an unexpected and severe breakdown. Hook (1963), in his study on 294 Swedish women who were refused abortion, did not find one single case of suicide or attempted suicide, though one-tenth made a threat of taking their own lives.[6]

The Social Argument

The medical and psychological arguments, while perhaps valid for a few, have, in general, been mainly a prelude to the clamour for abortion on demand: a social solution to a social problem. Again, the case was initially advanced with the support of heart-rending and dreadful case histories of young girls inconveniently pregnant and in seemingly desperate social situations. From there the push developed towards the concept that each pregnancy must be a wanted and planned event and that pregnancy outside such limits is a tyranny to be disposed of. Finally, and predictably, the position developed where it is argued that it is the right of the woman in question, in all circumstances, to retain or dispose of a pregnancy if she chooses without the wishes of any other party being taken into consideration. The vast majority of abortions are now carried out for social reasons, although it not infrequently happens that the social worker gets support from a psychiatrist.

In general, it has been made explicit in most abortion legislation that abortion remains a crime unless it is carried out under certain circumstances. The laws are usually so formed that many interpretations can be placed on them and *de facto* abortion on demand is available, especially if there is money to pay for it.

The Risks of Abortion

In general, I am against debates concerning the safety or otherwise of induced abortion, especially when conducted by non-medical persons. A willingness to enter into more than superficial debate can seem to give tacit approval to the whole concept of abortion, implying that only minor issues concerning it remain to be solved. For those committed to the pro-life movements it should not, as regards their strength of opposition to abortion, matter greatly whether abortion was made as safe as brushing one's teeth or cleaning one's nails. However, some discussion as to the hazards is appropriate.

The medical literature during the past decade abounds with papers extolling the safety of various techniques of abortion and with many papers annotating the lists of hazards and complications.[7] Much caution must be exercised in interpreting all these reports and certainly they must be treated with a greater reserve than is usually appropriate to scientific literature. This is because most of the papers are produced by workers with a very definite ideology (one might say prejudice) and in these circumstances separating the objective from the subjective data can be virtually impossible.

In general terms the earlier the abortion is carried out the less damage both physically and psychologically. However, performed by whatever technique abortion does endanger the mother in four general ways; trauma, infection, haemorrhage and psychologically. Death of the mother is also a sequela of induced abortion, though this is a rare occurrance. In 1978 in the United States eleven women died following legally induced abortions (US Department of Health and Human Services Report).

Trauma. Damage to the uterus may lead to haemorrhage, shock and occasionally to death. Tears in the cervix may lead to problems of spontaneous miscarriage in subsequent pregnancies. There have been reports, albeit rarely, of damage to the bowel, bladder and even to large blood vessels.

Haemorrhage. Again, the uterus may bleed due to trauma or to its inability to contract. The patient's blood may not coagulate, resulting in profound haemorrhage. If a mother is rhesus negative, abortion may be associated with a transfusion syndrome with all the possible disease sequelae.

Infection. Post-abortal sepsis is always a risk no matter how 'perfectly' the abortion is performed. The further the situation is from 'perfect' the greater will be the problem. In situations of poor sterility, bacteremic shock can be a serious and occasionally fatal problem.

The psychological sequelae are less tangible and have already, to a certain extent, been discussed.

The Opposition to Abortion and the Growth of Pro-Life

The decade since the introduction of liberal abortion legislation in many western countries has also seen the growth of many and often vociferous pro-life movements. These have often been, but not always, closely linked with the Roman Catholic Church. For the often confused layman living in an age of at least expressed ecumenism, there is no doubt that the absolute rejection of abortion is one of the chief divergences in ethical thinking between Catholics and other Christian denominations. While other Christians may hesitate, the Catholic consensus is maintained and dialogue tends to be minimal.

The Roman Church, while always maintaining its stance against abortion, has varied in the expression of its opposition from a studied silence to the use of language that ensures that only those deeply committed to the anti-abortion movement will listen.

In 1973 Cardinal Heenan confessed that during the debate on the new legislation in Britain, Catholics had committed a strategic mistake: 'The Catholic Church deliberately made no pronouncement against the Abortion Bill because we were told that if Catholics did so it would confirm the humanist argument that only Catholics object to abortion. We now all know what a terrible thing that abortion law is.'

Conversely much Catholic opposition to abortion both publicly and in private has been formed in words and phrases that ensure no prospect of reasoned debate. One only has to think of the rhetorical overkill in which Catholic propagandists frequently indulge. By that I mean the use of language that makes it quite impossible for their opponents ever to listen to them. Talk of mass murder, genocide, massacre of the innocents, and invoking memories of the Third Reich, while perhaps understandable, cannot begin to convince the opposition and alienates the middle ground. The argument disappears in the emotiveness and reason loses out.

The Society for the Protection of the Unborn Child was formed as a non-denominational society to protect the foetus, to publicise the facts about abortion, and to exert as much political muscle as possible to try and change the law in the United Kingdom.

Another organisation termed 'Life' grew up in the United Kingdom and it now also has offices in Ireland. It is affiliated to the International Pro-Life Movement and to Life Line. 'Life' is non-denominational and non-party-political. It is exclusively anti-abortion and wants laws permitting abortion repealed. 'Life' gives pregnancy-testing services, counselling and immediate positive and practical help to all women and girls regardless of age, marital status, creed, race, etc. who have unplanned or problem pregnancies. The service, provided by trained, volunteer personnel, is designed to enable a woman with pregnancy problems fully to discuss her situation and to get help throughout pregnancy and for as long after birth as necessary so that she may avoid abortion. 'Life' arranges accommodation before and after birth for those made homeless by pregnancy or who wish to move as a result of pregnancy. Baby-sitting services, baby clothes and equipment are provided as required. 'Life' exists to help solve problems created by pregnancy without harming the mother or her child.

The Only Argument

I come now to what I feel represent the only real arguments against abortion, which, I believe, if advanced in a sympathetic spirit, free of sermonising or hectoring, and in language likely to be listened to, will in the end be the most successful.

There is, in my judgment, not much to be gained from invoking theological principles in arguing against abortion. This is because, powerful as arguments concerning God as the creator of us all may be, they are for real use amongst theists and believers. Principles of discussion requiring a belief in God have little sense when used with people who do not, themselves, share belief in God as Creator or, indeed, hold a Christian view. Moreover, and regrettably, those who do show fundamental tenets of Christian belief can come to very different views on abortion. The report on the Anglican Working Party is not untypical. '. . .This (justification of abortion) would be when at the request of the mother and after the kind of consultation which we have envisaged in the report, it could be established that there was a threat to the mother's life or well-being and hence inescapably to her health, if she were obliged to carry the child to term and give it birth.'[8] Not all Anglicans would agree. Far from it. But this report reminds us that amongst the most devout and formal of Christians there is a spectrum of viewpoints.

Therefore, I feel that the arguments against abortion should be conducted from a philosophical rather than a theological basis. This does not mean simply arguing from first principles or dealing only in abstractions. Still less does it mean neglecting the evidence from medical or sociological sources. Rather it means collating all these clues or pieces of evidence and incorporating them into an ever developing treatise on the nature of the foetus. It means asking the right questions, on the right level and in the correct order. This approach could offer a very real service to the whole pluralist community which, quite literally, has little knowledge of what it is doing when it says either 'yes' or 'no' to abortion. It also could demonstrate that it is possible to be opposed to something and have good reasons for being so opposed.

I feel that as a start we should break down the question concerning the status of the foetus into four compartments and use every piece of evidence; physiological, medical, psychological and sociological to answer them. We therefore should ask:

Is the foetus alive?
Is the foetus individual and distinct?
Is the foetus human?
Is the foetus a person?

Is the Foetus Alive? This is by far the easiest of the four questions. It can be readily shown from the earliest time following conception that cellular growth is taking place at a phenomenal rate. In fact, at the time most abortions take place pretty well every adult bodily function is taking place with the exception of breathing and perhaps mentation. The foetus certainly feels pain at this stage and therefore undoubtedly feels the pain associated with its termination.

Is the Foetus Individual? This is most important as many of the advocates of abortion relegate the foetus to a type of maternal appendage which can be chopped off or out when not desired. It is claimed that the mother has rights over her own body and, therefore, has the right to dispose of what is a temporary part of it: her foetus. The whole problem, of course, of self-mutilation is another day's debate but in any case it cannot validly be applied to the foetus. Even taking into account the obvious symbiotic relationship between a mother and her foetus, medical science shows us that the foetus is genetically and biologically clearly distinct from its mother. In fact, why the mother does not reject her foetus as a foreign series of proteins in a similar fashion to the way she might reject an incompatible blood transfusion or a transplanted kidney remains a major and essentially unsolved mystery to immunologists. It is a subject being intensely researched – often, paradoxically, by reproductive scientists who passionately favour abortion on the grounds of the mother having total dominion over her own body. The foetus very often has a separate blood group from its mother and their bloods never normally admix.

The foetus has its own identifiable finger-prints and its heart beats at a different rate to its mother's. The genetic coding of the foetus is totally distinct. Certainly the foetus is totally dependant on its mother but then which of us is not dependant on someone else or on a group of persons for our continued existence. If the question of independent survival comes up, as it does, it can only be stated and stated clearly that few if any of us can independently survive. Yes, the foetus is clearly an individual.

Is the Foetus Human? This problem is difficult to resolve in any simple way. Certainly the DNA coding of the foetus is human, its proteins are human, it can only become a human, it cannot become anything else. The potentiality of the foetus, as that of the new-born baby, is to develop into an adult human. There is no known biological time, either before or after birth, when a definite sudden change takes place. Life is all a continuum, and as towards the end one does not cease to be human, there is similarly no obvious start, except at the time of conception. The often cited difference between human and humanised life and the theory of society's acceptance of the full measure of human life may exercise the minds of psychologists and sociologists. It has little relevance for the medical scientist.

Is the Foetus a Person? Again, this is not one really for the medical scientist. Psychologists can bring in concepts of when is a person, the necessity of achievement, the acceptance by contemporary society and so on. Again, while not meaning to be dismissive, the arguments about this, because of their necessary abstraction, are usually lost on the biologist and medical scientist and if in any way valid could probably be applied almost equally to those in post-natal life, with all the potential and appalling consequences.

Therefore, I feel that from sheer reason, backed by science, it should be obvious that the foetus is a living individual human being and by deduction entitled to all the care and protection usually afforded by contemporary society to its own kind. To argue otherwise represents discrimination, a type of prenatal apartheid and one that is more vicious than any of the usually discussed oppressions or apartheid, for it attacks and discriminates against those most utterly defenceless who are not even given the pretence of advocacy on their behalf.

Of course, the above arguments would be laughed out by many committed abortionists because of their necessary abstraction. Well worked out philosophical concepts have little relevance to the girl in trouble. This is probably true, but it does not invalidate the arguments. It perhaps should only remind us that decisions taken in times of crises are not necessarily the best or the most enduring.

This is where we can help. The more we oppose abortion, the more we ought to show compassion and understanding to those who seek it. We should dispense with the abstract compassion of pious sentiments and indulge more in practical compassion of action. We must remember that the request for abortion is very often, and paradoxically, a plea for life, the mother's own life, her family's, her career opportunities, her concept of the poor lifestyle she could offer her baby, etc. Therefore, we should be pro-life rather than anti-abortion. We should show by action that there is an alternative, that there is help that can result in a full life for both and that the lonely journey of a rejected person can in many instances be avoided. This means work. Words are easy. The pro-life movement which offers refuge and time to a girl inconveniently pregnant must be encouraged, funded and supported. In this, and only in this way will we make abortion as unnecessary as possible.

4

Psychological Aspects of Termination of Pregnancy

NOEL WALSH

Cure her of that:
Cans't thou not minister to a mind diseas'd;
Pluck from the memory a rooted sorrow;
Raze out the written troubles of the brain;
And with some sweet oblivious antidote
Cleanse the stuff'd bosom of that perilous stuff
Which weights upon the heart.

(*Macbeth*)

The orientation of this article is based on psychotherapy with women seeking psychological help following termination of pregnancy. For many such women the major psychological task is coming to terms with a 'rooted sorrow'. In discussing this issue I attempt to bring together concepts and ideas derived from a variety of areas in modern psychoanalytic and psychological research, particularly those of attachment, grief, psychic numbing and psychotherapy.

Attachment Behaviour

One of the most fundamental concepts in understanding human relationships is that of attachment behaviour. This refers to the human tendency, also observed in animals, to form an affectionate bond with a mothering figure, or her substitute. This can usually be observed during the first year of life and the process is one in which the infant differentiates the mother from other persons in its environment and shows a marked preference to interact with her. This tendency to recognise the mother, to prefer her presence to that of others, is a particular feature of the mother/child interaction in the first two or three years of life. In a normal relationship the mother responds positively to the various behavioural patterns manifested by her child. She will feed in hunger, soothe in pain and comfort in distress. This gives the child a basic sense of security and creates a base from which it begins to express its curiosity and need to explore the environment. As the child matures it develops a capacity to form attachments to other persons, such as father, other siblings, and favoured non-animate objects, such as toys and other personal possessions. Other components which can be observed in the attachment process are the expression of strong feelings towards the mother, ranging from affection, pleasure and satisfaction to frustration and rage. These early patterns of feelings and relationships tend to be enduring even though they will undergo progressive modification as the child matures.

The mother/child relationship may be impaired by such factors as maternal rejection of the child. This may be overt because of the mother's inherent difficulty in fulfilling the maternal role, or due to illness, either physical or psychiatric in nature, such as depression or other adverse circumstances in the mother's life. It is in such circumstances that the earliest manifestations of human anxiety and depression related to disturbed attachment can be observed. Other factors tending to create anxiety in this early stage are discontinuities of the mother/child relationship caused by repeated absences of the mother, or separations related to frequent hospitalisations of either mother or infant, marital disharmony, separation or divorce. There is a great range and variety of family disruptions which may lead to real or threatened separation of this kind with their associated separation anxiety.

John Bowlby, using data from his own research and that of others, describes separation anxiety in some detail, and considers it a fundamental concept in understanding human distress, not only in infants and children, but throughout the life cycle. He describes three basic phases: protest – when the child misses the mother it gives expression to a mixture of tears, anger and hope that she will return. Next comes despair as she fails to reappear, and at this stage the earliest features of human grief and mourning can be observed as the child becomes quiet, sad and withdrawn. This painful state is followed by detachment – the child seems to forget the mother and becomes indifferent to her absence. Should she return he may appear not to recognise her or take any personal interest in her efforts to re-establish their relationship. Detachment can be considered a psychological defence mechanism to minimise or exclude the pain of separation and loss, and we will return to this later when we discuss the concept of psychic numbing.

Identification

Another important concept in understanding human relationships, which parallels that of attachment, is that of Identification. A distinction should be made between identification and imitation. In imitation the individual makes a personal and conscious effort to 'become like' another admired, loved or perhaps stronger person. However, the concept of identification implies a process which is unconscious and begins in infancy with the infant assimilating the behaviour, feelings and attitudes of its attachment figures, much as it takes in carbohydrates, proteins and fats in the nutritional sense. It is by first of all becoming attached to the mother and father and then identifying with them that the infant becomes like 'Mummy and Daddy'. Where the relationship between parent and child is charged with tension or hostility, the child may absorb a negative identification: 'I do not want to be like my hateful Mummy or Daddy.' It is important to recognise that identification tends to follow the relationship with attachment figures, and becomes increasingly selective as the infant, and later the child, differentiates himself from these key figures. This is the process whereby the earliest sense of self emerges.

A very important component of this sense of self is related to identification with the parent of the same or opposite sex. The young girl, as she differentiates herself from her mother or father, recognises that while she loves both parents, she is going to grow up and become female like her mother, and no matter how much she admires her father and wants to be like him, there is a fundamental recognition that this will not be possible. Likewise, the young boy may show a special affection and interest in his mother, but also recognises that he will not grow up to be like her, but like his father. It is important at this stage in development that the parent of the opposite sex positively affirms the value of the child's psychosexual identity. It is important that the father responds positively to the emerging femininity in his young daughter, so that her sense of becoming a young woman will first of all be related to her affection and identification with her mother, and secondly be affirmed in a positive way by her father. The young boy, who first of all is attached to and identified with his mother, and later with his father, seeks affirmation of his emerging masculinity from his mother. This process is a complex one and will be affected by the mother's attitude to her own femininity, her attitudes to being a wife and mother, her relationship with her husband and other men, which can be traced back to her own childhood relationships with her parents. Concurrently with this psychosexual differentiation in the process of attachment and identification, there is a wide range of personal qualities and characteristics in each parent with which the child may identify and assimilate as part of his or her personality. Many historical, cultural and social factors will influence particular aspects of psychosexual identity. In this century one important influence on the theory of female psychology has been psychoanalysis. Freud based his theory on clinical work and postulated that very early the young girl, recognising her differences from the male child, experienced feelings of anatomical deficiency, giving her a negative self-image of femininity. This theory is referred to as 'the genital trauma' theory. However, more recent work, particularly that of Erik Erikson, has emphasised a more positive aspect of female psychosexual identity. He introduces the concept of 'the valuable productive inner space.' Essentially what

Erikson is saying is that quite early in life the female child recognises that being female also means having the capacity to be a mother and give birth, something also recognised by the male child as a differentiating factor in his own psychosexual identification. Thus we see that these twin processes of attachment and identification, which occur throughout infancy, childhood and adolescence, play a major role in the capacity to form relationships with other people and give each person representational models of other significant people in their lives, and of their own selves.

As we follow these components of attachment and identification observed in the earliest relationship with the parents, we see them appearing again in adolescence as psychosexual maturity evolves. The young adolescent boy or girl manifests in relation to the opposite sex a need to attach to a particular individual. This individual is differentiated, selected and preferred to others, and is the object of strong feelings of affection associated with the anticipation of enduring relationship. These attachment feelings at this stage are linked to the emerging needs for intimacy and fidelity. Likewise, as the young adolescent woman develops, we can observe the evolution of the human capacity to nurture, to become a mother. This capacity contains the same essential psychological components already described in her previous stages of development and coming to fruition in the birth of her child with the emergence of spontaneous affection, an intense order of preference, and the capacity for an enduring relationship between mother and child. Thus we can see that a connecting thread exists between each individual's early experience with mother and father, and that attachment and identification throughout infancy, childhood and adolescence prepares each individual to be a parent in his or her own turn.

The Psychology of Pregnancy

If, then, we accept this approach to the psychology of woman, it would appear that once she recognises that she is pregnant, a process of attachment begins. At the beginning of pregnancy this capacity for attachment to her baby may not reach the level of personal consciousness, but gradually does so as the pregnancy proceeds and she begins to have feelings, fantasies and fears concerning her future child.

It would appear from clinical observation that this capacity for maternal attachment, or maternal feeling, varies in degree in different women, and will be related to the many complex developmental factors already outlined. Some women may have a basic deficiency in the capacity for maternal feeling, and attachment will not develop either during the pregnancy, or later. Perhaps we can speak of a progression from latent to fulfilled motherhood in the completion of pregnancy and the birth of a child. Many factors will influence maternal feelings and most important is the relationship with the father of her child. This can range from a relationship which is in essence based on an assault as in the case of rape, to one in which the father is deeply loved. In a situation where the relationship with the father has been that of an assault, or one in which there has been much conflict, hostility or abuse, the baby may be experienced as a hostile intrusion, and her maternal feelings be intermingled with negative images of the father.

The next type of relationship with the father could be broadly described as 'neutral'. By this I mean that she does not have particularly strong feelings of affection or hostility towards him. Such pregnancies may be related to sexual ignorance, naïvety, or lack of knowledge of the normal physiological processes of intercourse, conception and pregnancy. Other pregnancies may reflect the unconscious need to solve problems such as loneliness, depression, conflict regarding psychosexual identity, or possibly rebellion against unaccepted parental and personal moral or social values. Clinical experience indicates that in certain pregnancies the presence of hostile or neutral feelings towards the father may facilitate the suppression of maternal feelings or attachment. By contrast, the inner psychological situation of the woman appears different where she has strong affection or love for the father of her child. This may include a range of relationships from the unmarried mother to a happy marital situation, or extend to extra-marital relationships. It is in the context of a loving relationship that we see the positive and creative side of the maternal capacity and the need to have a baby.

Love, of its nature, tends to be enduring. The woman pregnant and carrying the child of a man she loves cannot see termination as the simple solution to what is an ongoing, fulfilling relationship, even if it takes place in the context of complex moral and social circumstances. However, in such a loving relationship the birth of a child can be perceived as a serious threat to the ongoing relationship, and in such circumstances some women may decide to 'sacrifice the pregnancy' rather than risk losing their relationship with the man they love. If this relationship should subsequently break down the woman is then faced with a double loss. This motive of sacrificing the pregnancy to preserve not only a loving relationship with the man, but also perhaps to preserve the psychological and personal wellbeing of a family, may be observed in situations where a woman is informed that she is carrying a damaged foetus, and is terrified at the consequences of giving birth to a handicapped child, and of having to take care of its upbringing in what may be difficult and adverse family circumstances.

So far, I have highlighted some of the factors in relationships which may facilitate the expression or suppression of attachment feelings towards the baby. There are, however, other important basic needs and feelings associated with the experience of pregnancy and giving birth to a child. These can best be considered as needs for continuity and creativity. Continuity is basically a need to achieve a sense of personal survival and immortality, and one of the most fundamental modes of fulfilling this need is the birth of a child and becoming a parent. This gives a sense of generational continuity from ancestors to one's children's children. This is described as biological continuity. Closely linked with this need for continuity is a need for creativity. While this may find its expression in a great range of human activities, giving birth to a child is a uniquely feminine capacity and experience, and would appear to be related to fundamental forms of feminine fulfilment and creativity. It appears that once the pregnancy is on its way the elements of attachment, continuity and creativity, however unconscious or latent, come into action and seek their fulfilment in the ongoing process of pregnancy and the birth of a child.

It has been observed that when a woman spontaneously loses the baby not only may she experience giref at the time of the loss, but may also have feelings of depression at the time the baby would have been born. The deep sense of loss experienced by women who give birth to stillborn infants is further evidence of the importance of these elements in the process of pregnancy. Erikson reports from his clinical observations that there are specific forms of loneliness and depression related to the active inner space in women, which do not occur in men.

So far we have examined relationships between the mother and her baby and the father of her child. It may now be of value to examine her relationships with her family and the broader community in which she participates. The social circumstances in which a pregnant woman finds herself vary enormously, and include such factors as age, state of health, economic circumstances, marital status and the presence or absence of psychological, social and religious support. It is important to emphasise that many of these complex forces are going to operate either positively or negatively towards making a decision within a very short space of time, usually a matter of weeks, since the woman is normally four to six weeks pregnant at the time of confirmation of her pregnancy. Psychologically, she is attempting to compress complex psychobiological experience, which normally takes nine months, into a matter of weeks, or sometimes days. In these stressful circumstances it is necessary to explore other relationships which may be available to a woman in helping her to make a decision. Here we have to examine her life situation and social network. If there is a supportive family relationship, the attitudes taken by her parents, other members of her family, close friends in whom she may confide, will play an important role in her decision. Some women with religious convictions may seek direction from their spiritual advisers, yet others will consult their family doctor. Those who have a particular type of work, or aspire to a special career, may see this as an influential factor in their decision. The social philosophy of the particular society in which a woman lives may be an important influence in terms of the pressure it brings on her to have a termination, or, alternatively, in the support systems, both psychological and economic, which it provides to help her in favour of her pregnancy. In certain societies there is a significant investment in encouraging the woman to continue her pregnancy and social, financial and psychological support for the woman is provided, with the expectation that following the birth of her child, this child will be given in adoption. There are both moral and psychological and indeed existential implications in this approach in that, first of all, from the moral point of view the rights of the foetus are regarded as having priority. Psychologically it reflects a tradition in which the woman is regarded as having a more positive and self-affirming experience in giving birth than in terminating her pregnancy. While giving full importance to these moral and psychological principles, it is important also to recognise that the process of adoption involves important psychological problems for both the mother and the child. It is essential to recognise that adoption as a solution involves a permanent severance of the maternal attachment of the woman to her child, while the child, at a later stage, as it becomes aware of its role as an adoptee, will have to make its own important psychological adjustments. This raises the issue of the provision of adequate support systems in the post-adoption situation. Ultimately, whatever choice the woman makes, be it in favour of her pregnancy and adoption, or of termination, suffering will be inevitable. An increasing number of women now decide to keep their child and live in a one-parent family situation.

Unfortunately, many women who find themselves pregnant do not have the support of a personal family, or close friends, and may be living in relative social isolation or extreme poverty. They may not have access to whatever resources the particular community has to offer and such women will often be left to make their decisions in isolation.

We have now examined a number of influences affecting the woman's decision-making process, and not least will be that of the father of the child, who, after all, is more than an internalised psychological relationship. He is also an individual who may or may not take a definite stand towards the birth of a child. His support, or lack of it, for the pregnancy will be a critical factor as she tries to make her decision. In some instances the woman may decide not to inform the father of her child that she is pregnant. In other words, the knowledge that he is the father of the child, and the affirmation of his potency, and the awakening of his capacity for fatherhood, and the degree of responsibility he may be willing to take, are dependent on the woman's attitude towards him, and the degree to which she accepts or allows his involvement.

It appears, then, in the concrete situation in which a woman finds herself pregnant in adverse circumstances, she has to balance a complex series of relationships, such as her own maternal needs, her relationship with the father of her child, the presence or absence of family support, her relationship to work and career, her personal moral and religious convictions, and the social philosophy of the society in which she is living.

In making a choice to terminate the woman will usually seek final sanction with the medical profession. This may be a personal or family doctor, possibly a psychiatrist, or she may consult with the gynaecologist whom she requests to perform the act of termination itself. It is at this stage that the medical profession begins to share in the responsibility for the procedures which are going to be undertaken. The setting, atmosphere and relationship formed with the medical staff performing the termination procedure, may play an important part in the woman's perception of the experience, and affect to a significant degree her subsequent feelings and reactions to the event.

Pregnancy in Adversity

Statistics available from different parts of the world indicate that an increasing number of women in a wide range of circumstances react to pregnancy and perceived adversity by making a decision to terminate. Having examined the deep and complex emotions involved in the experience of pregnancy, and the variety of pressures towards termination as a solution, one must ask what, if any, psychological damage occurs from this interaction of forces, both internal and external. Follow-up studies on the psychological impact of termination have not reported any significant psychiatric illness. The question of the methodology and time span measurements of these follow-up studies raise fundamental questions about the nature of scientific enquiry into complex psychological experience. The observations in this article are based on clinical experience with women seeking psychological help following termination. It is important to make a distinction between the woman who has a spontaneous abortion (a miscarriage) who may be described as *losing* something whether it is accepted or rejected, and the woman who has a termination and thus has something *taken away* from her, again whether it is accepted or rejected. The woman who decides to terminate in effect hands herself and her potential child over to the medical profession and its technology. What is shared by both of these experiences is loss, but the sense of personal responsibility for what has happened is of a distinctly different psychological order.

Grief and Mourning

The normal psychological reaction to loss is grief and mourning. Tolstoy, in *War and Peace*, compares grief to a wound and mourning to the healing process. Most people would probably accept that termination can be considered a wound to the natural biological process of pregnancy, and if the intricate network of psychological relationships accompanying this process, as already outlined, is accepted, then this wound or disruption must have psychological consequences. In following the analogy of wound and healing to grief and mourning, it is important to emphasise not only the concept of damage, but also that of the healing process. Just as recovering from a wound requires healing, so recovery from a loss requires mourning. Where grief takes place overtly, it will be accompanied by acute distress, painful moods of anguish and sadness, crying spells, perhaps insomnia and a preoccupation with the stressful event. Gradually, over a period of time, which will vary with the nature of the loss, and the internal and external resources available to the person, a working through of the mourning process will take place. However, in many circumstances grief and mourning do not automatically occur, and the experience of loss is frequently suppressed; just as in the physical order it is instinctive to withdraw from physical pain, likewise it is psychologically protective to withdraw from psychological pain, and here we come to the concept of psychological defence. One of the basic defence mechanisms in psychologically stressful situations is that of closing off of feeling which is referred to as 'psychic numbing', or 'emotional anaesthesia'. It is the psychological equivalent of withdrawing or protecting oneself from physical pain. We described an earlier manifestation of defence in discussing the detachment of the child when the mother fails to return after repeated or prolonged absences. Psychic numbing appears to be the mechanism by which all the complex and painful feelings which surround the decision to terminate and its aftermath are closed off, and may explain why so many women who have this experience have no overt feelings at the time, or for some time afterwards. It may also be a reason why many studies fail to identify depression or other adverse psychological sequelae. What is being measured is the psychological experience of women who are using this defence mechanism and are not consciously reporting any psychological or somatic distress. However, clinical experience suggests that psychological defence mechanisms do not contain painful conflict or loss indefinitely, and that they continue to seek expression as so well stated by Shakespeare:

> Give sorrow words,
> Grief that does not speak,
> Whispers to the o'erfraught heart
> And bids it break.
>
> (*Macbeth*)

Modern studies of psychic numbing indicate that individuals going through this experience may not show any overt psychiatric symptomatology, or even necessarily complain of depression, but will have a certain form of inner psychological constriction, loss of vitality, and a sense of not being fully in contact with all their deeper feelings and personal experience. Sometimes they report episodes of crying, or moods of sadness. One woman in her forties whose only pregnancy had been terminated, reported 'At times I feel an inexpressible sorrow.' Clinical experience with women who have had terminations suggests that these constrictions are focused on the inner psychological areas of maternal feelings, and female sexuality. What psychological impact this focused constriction will have on a woman's relationship with existing or subsequent children raises some very interesting and unexplored psychological issues.

Guilt feelings appear to be an intrinsic component of grief and mourning. Normal guilt is related to a sense of having transgressed a particular rule or law. Usually there is a proportion between the amount of guilt experienced and the degree of transgression committed. This will vary with the personal, social and religious upbringing of each woman. Some will consider termination as an assault of the inviolable right to life of the foetus, and a serious personal offence against God's ultimate authority – others will not. In the former it can be expected that guilt feelings, often severe, will occur, and can be regarded as a proportionate psychological reaction to a perceived serious transgression of an objective moral code. Self-condemnation, the need for forgiveness and atonement, are part of a normal sequence of psychological reactions. Such women, particularly those with a Catholic or Christian background, may seek forgiveness for what they regard as a serious sin through the Sacrament of Confession. The experience of forgiveness mediated through the Church and the personal confessor will be of great help to many. However, the need to assimilate the experience of termination at the psychological level will be an ongoing problem in terms of loss and guilt feelings which will not be removed by confession and which have their source in the developmental history of the individual. It is of interest to note that many women who do not perceive termination as an objective moral transgression will also experience guilt feelings. These guilt feelings appear to be related to fundamental human experiences bound up with the fact that the termination occurred at a particular time which is now irreversible, that it has an ultimate finality, and that no action on the woman's part can bring about the recovery, or the potential, of what has been lost or taken away.

Not all guilt feelings are proportionate to a sense of personal transgression of an accepted moral law. Normal guilt feelings are associated with the need to set the balance right, to repay a debt, to atone. In this connection it is interesting that Ekblad, in a study of Swedish women who had terminations, described the phenomenon of the atonement child as a tendency for the woman to become pregnant again within two years. By contrast, abnormal or neurotic guilt feelings are characterised by a sense that the debt can never be repaid or the damage undone. This may lead to a repetitive pattern of self-blame and condemnation.

Another important characteristic of abnormal guilt feelings is that the individual may condemn herself as severely for *wishing* to transgress her personal rules as if she had actually done so. This can be frequently observed in relation to aggressive and hostile feelings, and appears to explain the guilt feelings observed following the loss of a relationship or an attachment in which there appears to be no basis for guilt feelings, and the relationship has been positive and affectionate. This can be explained on the basis that all attachment relationships, however harmonious, involve some degree of frustration, anger and hostility, hence the tendency to a disproportionate reaction, even in the normal situation.

In many women who have terminations these complex and painful feelings of guilt, together with those of loss, will be excluded from consciousness and appear not significant in psychological or somatic terms, and remain unexpressed for months or years. Many women will regard termination as an entirely private and personal event, which has not been traumatic, and has never been considered an important aspect of their life history; these do not seek any form of therapy. Other women because of their distress may seek help at the time or immediately after the termination.

Psychotherapy

The present writer's experience is in the field of medical psychotherapy, and what follows is an outline of some of the factors which appear important in helping women who seek some resolution of the experience of termination. Essentially the therapist is one who presents himself or herself as a person with professional training who wishes to help the woman with this particular problem. It is essential that the therapist be *non-judgmental* and have sufficient experience and training so that his or her own personal attitudes do not intrude into the atmosphere of moral freedom, sympathetic understanding and tolerance that a good therapeutic relationship requires. This non-judgmental attitude is entirely compatible with the therapist having his or her own moral values concerning the nature of termination. Even when the therapist is non-judgmental, as therapy proceeds it is normal for the patient to perceive him in terms of pre-existing models of significant attachment figures, invariably parental. Thus the therapist may be perceived as caring or not caring, condemning or forgiving. It is essential to recognise the distortions and disproportions in these images which a patient forms of the therapist. Where a woman turns to a spiritual adviser, personal counsellor or other significant helper, many of the same factors will operate, and will need to be recognised and understood. As the patient reviews her life and the stressful circumstances in which her decision to terminate was made, she will have an opportunity to work through her complex feelings which to date have been suppressed by psychic numbing. It is in this process, usually involving months or longer, that she has an opportunity to express her feelings of loss, guilt, anger and the many factors influencing her decision. Many therapeutic sessions may centre around questions of moral and ethical values. It is important to make a distinction between one's moral and personal ethical development. We can speak of a primitive morality developing during infancy and childhood, when the earliest do's and don'ts of the parents are internalised. It brings us back to the early identification process where what one should or should not do is absorbed with one's attachment to one's parents. This primitive morality is based on the fear of punishment and the withdrawal of love. It is on the foundation of this primitive morality that one's personal ethical values emerge as one matures through the different stages of infancy, childhood and adolescence into adult life. This distinction between the morality of childhood and the evolution of personal ethical values will inevitably be confronted in the therapeutic situation. In this process many of the primitive feelings related to fear of punishment and withdrawal of love will be directed to the therapist as a representational model of the original attachment figures.

In some women their childhood experience was to be punished for wrong doing by a parent who could not easily forgive. Such parents may have consistently failed to distinguish between the offending action and its motives and have thereby induced a sense of personal unworthiness in the child which can persist into adolescence and adult life. If this pattern occurs in childhood it will be accompanied by a feeling of isolation and inner constriction in relation to any action the child considers 'bad behaviour'. It does not give the child the essential learning experience that guilt is not only personal but interpersonal. A simple example could be that of the child who breaks a window while playing and is made to feel not only that he has transgressed a parental prohibition, but also has no possibility *on his own* of repairing the damage. This highlights not only the sense of personal responsibility for what has happened, but also the parental response which may vary from the closed and punitive to the open, understanding and forgiving. In the closed parental response the child is offered no possibility for atonement, and this may encourage him to deny or conceal what has occurred.

Returning to the therapeutic situation we can see that a woman with an expectation of a closed parental response will not perceive the therapist as a person who will be open, understanding and forgiving, at the psychological level. One of the major tasks of therapy will be to help the woman to understand and work through this pattern of inflexibility in her own life. In doing this one of the dangers for the therapist is to feel that he may also forgive her at the moral level, and here once again it becomes important to distinguish between guilt at the psychological level and that arising from the woman's awareness of having transgressed a personal ethical value. In therapeutic practice one frequently observes that for many women it is only by working through this childhood level of morality that the possibility of more freely examining and searching for their own ethical values is reached. In the context of termination, these values will usually centre around such issues as the personhood of the foetus, and the injury inflicted on it, the relationship with the father, one's relationship to one's own continuity and creativity and ultimately, in those who believe in God, a personal reconciliation, including with her own child in heaven, and hopefully a recognition that the self is not closed but moves forward in time to new possibilities.

Acknowledgment. I would like to thank Dr Mary Darby, Consultant Psychiatrist, St Vincent's Hospital, for her helpful discussion on many of the points outlined in this article.

5

The Treatment of Infertility: Ethical Issues

NIALL DUIGNAN

Approximately one in every ten marriages is associated with infertility. It is now apparent that identifiable male factors contribute significantly in 35 to 40 per cent of infertile marriages, so it is important to stress that any investigation of infertility implies an investigation of an infertile couple and not simply an infertile wife as frequently occurred in the past. This chapter gives a brief summary of the causes, investigation and treatment of inferility followed by a more detailed consideration of ethical problems that may arise in relation to different forms of therapy.

Causes of Infertility

In the female, infertility may be due to (i) failure of ovulation, (ii) failure of the ova to reach the uterus due to a blockage in the fallopian tubes, sometimes termed the oviduct, or (iii) a reaction between the cervical mucus – the mucus secreted by the glands in the neck of the womb – and the husband's sperm.

In the male, infertility is mainly due to (i) defects in coital techniques, such as impotence or the use of lubricants during intercourse, (ii) abnormalities of testicular function, (iii) an obstruction to the passage of sperm, or (iv) some abnormality in the prostate or seminal vesicles.

In addition to the causes listed above, psychosexual problems affecting either the husband or wife may give rise to infertility. On the male side the psychosexual problems are likely to give rise to impotence or premature ejaculation, and on the female side to cause vaginismus. When psychosexual problems are present, it is important that the couple should be referred for joint therapy to a person trained in such matters.

Investigations

The investigation of the infertile couple is aimed at attempting to discover if any abnormality of reproductive function exists so that definitive treatment may be given. It is important to realise that despite full investigation no definitive abnormality may be discovered.

In the female, failure of ovulation can be detected from a basal body temperature record kept by the patient, or by hormonal investigations. An obstruction in the fallopian tubes can be discovered by either taking a special X-ray or by the use of laparoscopy, which consists of inserting a telescope into the abdominal cavity and obtaining a direct view of the pelvic organs. An abnormality in the cervical mucus is detected by examining a patient during the middle of the menstrual cycle some hours after intercourse has taken place so that the mucus can be assessed and any reaction between sperm and mucus noted.

The investigation of the husband consists of a full examination, together with an assessment of the quality and quantity of sperm. The sperm may be assessed during a post-coital test which demonstrates any reaction between sperm and cervical mucus. Generally speaking, a good post-coital test implies that a sperm count is satisfactory. However, whenever a post-coital test is not normal, then there is no substitute for the adequate and careful evaluation of the husband's semen. This is the key investigation in the assessment of the infertile male. Semen should be collected by masturbation into a clean glass or plastic container with a non-metallic lid as contact with metal can inhibit sperm motility. Masturbation is preferred as a method of collection as the greatest concentration of sperm are released early in the ejaculatory process and this fraction can be lost if the sample is collected by *coitus interruptus*.[1] In some instances hormonal tests, chromosome analysis or testicular biopsies may be required to complete the investigation of the male, but these tests are usually only necessary when an abnormality in sperm count has previously been discovered.

Treatment

The infertile female, in whom infertility is due to failure of ovulation, can be readily treated with a variety of drugs with success rates of 80 to 90 per cent in some instances. Each woman has to be assessed individually and the appropriate endocrinological therapy given. The induction of ovulation with drugs does not present any ethical problems. Infertility due to a reaction between a wife's cervical mucus and her husband's sperm is difficult to treat effectively and such an abnormality may be found in up to 10 per cent of infertile couples in whom a definitive lesion is isolated. Women in whom a blockage of the fallopian tubes is found may respond to surgery in some instances, or be hopelessly sterile in others.

The treatment of the infertile male remains disappointing to date, no doubt due to our inadequate understanding of the problem. One exception to this is where a low sperm count is associated with the presence of a varicocele around the testes; in such instances removal of the varicocele may be followed by a significant increase in the number of sperms and subsequent fertility. Notwithstanding the poor results of treatment, all husbands should be carefully assessed, even though the outcome may establish the presence of irreversible sterility. Such an evaluation, however, can spare the patient and his wife considerable anxiety and prevent the far too frequent multiple consultation of doctors. Tact, compassion and explanation can help the sterile male to realise that his role as a husband is not compromised, despite sterility, thereby preventing needless strain on the marital unit.

Ethical Considerations

Ethical problems concerning the infertile couple arise when consideration is given to the investigation of the infertile male as well as when considering certain forms of medical therapy suitable for either the infertile male or female.

The main areas where ethical problems arise can be summarised under the following headings:

(i) collection of samples for seminal analysis;
(ii) artificial insemination with either husband or donor sperm;
(iii) *in vitro* fertilisation;
(iv) the foster womb;
(v) the artificial placenta.

Collection of Samples for Seminal Analysis. A sample of semen for seminal analysis may be obtained by withdrawal during intercourse at the time of ejaculation or by masturbation. The majority of medical opinion feels that a more satisfactory sample can be obtained by masturbation rather than by withdrawal. The ethical problems concerned with the collection of a semen sample by masturbation are the same as those which pertain to the collection of samples for artificial insemination with husband's sperm and are considered in detail in the following discussion.

Artificial Insemination. Artificial insemination is a relatively simple medical procedure which provides an alternative to sterility for some couples. It is performed by introducing semen via a syringe into the female vagina, cervical canal or uterus in order to induce pregnancy. The procedure has a high success rate in some instances, depending on such variables as the quality of semen specimen and the timing of insemination. There is no evidence of any increased abortion or abnormality rate in the progeny. There are two basic types of artificial insemination: homologous, when the semen is obtained from the husband (AIH); and heterologous, when the semen is acquired from a donor (AID).

Artificial insemination raises complex ethical and social issues as it alters the natural processes of procreation and provides human beings with potential for exercising control over the generation and quality of human life. AIH and AID raise separate ethical considerations and these should be considered separately.

AIH can be used to overcome physical or psychological difficulties which preclude cervical insemination through normal sexual intercourse. It can also be used in the management of some cases of oligospermia, i.e. a low sperm count, whereby a number of ejaculates are pooled so that the spermatozoa can be separated from the semen and subsequently inseminated in a concentrated form.

Within the Catholic Church, AIH was for years defended by some as at least probably permissible if semen was obtained in a licit and non-masturbatory way. However, in 1949, Pius XII intervened and said that AIH was to be absolutely eliminated. He spoke in more detail on this matter in 1951 as follows:

> To reduce the co-habitation of married persons and the conjugal act to a mere organic function for the transmission of the germ of life, would be to convert the domestic hearth, sanctuary of the family, into nothing more than a biological laboratory . . . The conjugal act in its natural structure is a personal action, a simultaneous natural self-giving which, in the words of Holy Scripture, effects the union in one flesh. This is more than the mere union of two germs, which can be brought about artificially, that is, without the natural action of the spouses. The conjugal act as it is planned and willed by nature, implies a personal co-operation, the right to which the parties have mutually conferred on each other in contracting marriage.[2]

The argument, then, of Pius XII was that AIH is immoral, because the child so born is not the fruit of an act which is itself expressive of personal love. Thus, the Pope's guidance seems to suggest that only intercourse between husband and wife properly expresses the personal procreative co-operation of parenthood.

Father J. Mahoney, S.J., has suggested in an article that perhaps marital intercourse was not the only possible method of creative married love.[3] The loving desire of a couple to have a child of their own, despite some difficulties on their part, might have some bearing on the clinical procedures condemned by the Pope. Their mutual love and their wish for a child might perhaps bring new light on the practice of obtaining semen by masturbation. Such a practice according to the traditional argument frustrates the purpose of procreation, yet in the case of AIH its use would appear to be for the sole purpose of procreation. Further, the objection that masturbation is a solitary expression of sexuality would not seem to hold, since in these circumstances it could be construed as an act by the husband out of loving concern for his wife and a desire on both their parts to produce a child of their marriage.

On the other hand, AID presents a totally different problem. Two forms of AID are practised: in one instance, samples of semen are obtained from suitable donors, frozen and kept in sperm banks until required; in the other form, fresh samples of sperm are obtained by masturbation from suitable donors and placed, within a few minutes, into the cervix or uterus.

Until recently the great majority of people considered AID appalling, but the attitudes of some have changed considerably in the past decade. However, within the Catholic community, there never was and still is not much wavering on AID, although occasionally individual authors manifest doubts or even endorse it as ethically acceptable. However, Catholics still see it as generally morally wrong for four main reasons: (i) it violates the marriage covenant; (ii) there is no bond of origin between the marriage partners and a child which is the fruit of the active element of a third person, even though the husband consents. Furthermore as Pius XII put it, nature imposes on whoever gives life to a small creature the task of its preservation and education; (iii) once conceded the right, even by their own husbands, to be inseminated artificially by the seed of another man, wives might too easily conclude that it would be preferable to receive seed in the natural way, i.e. by sexual intercourse; thus adulteries would be multiplied to the detriment of marriage. This seems more likely to occur when fresh semen samples are used for AID; (iv) the human stud farming mentality towards marriage would be fostered.

The selection of donors for AID in itself raises a number of ethical and social questions. Since the donor has no control over the use of his semen, responsibility for how the semen is used now rests with the physician. However, the nature and limits of his responsibility remain undefined. For example, what criteria should a physician use in selecting a 'suitable' donor? Are there minimal medical and genetic tests that should be conducted? Although there is a danger of transmitting infectious or genetic diseases through AID, present methods of donor selection and testing vary widely. Such differences mean that prospective recipients and the community have no minimum standards of practice upon which to rely.

A consent agreement between the recipient and the physician should be signed in all cases in order to protect the rights and welfare of all parties involved. The emotional effects of donor insemination, its ambiguous legal status and a possibility of transmitting infectious and genetic diseases are compelling reasons for obtaining informed consent. What information should such agreements include? Are recipients entitled to know the donor's health status and semen quality? Should they be given a genetic profile of the donor? The ethical and legal responsibilities of the physician performing AID to inform his patients remain unclear at the present time.

In addition to the factors mentioned above, AID creates the enormous problem of deciding what qualities should be bred and who should make the decisions. Some would use AID for the general improvement of the genetic pool with the formation of sperm banks comprised of frozen sperm from outstanding men and ovum banks with oocytes from outstanding women. The immediate question that this would pose is: is it justified to 'improve' the human race? A disproportionate use of certain donors would probably result in the eventual reduction of genetic variability in the entire population. It may therefore be morally and biologically unwise to tamper with human genes without greater knowledge regarding the conditions of future environments.

There has been little discussion of AID where the husband is fertile but the wife sterile. This would involve an anonymous donor to provide the husband his self fulfilment as a father. Such an action could occur in two manners: an anonymous donor could be impregnated with the husband's sperm in a manner similar to that used for artificial insemination with donor sperm, or a husband might have sexual intercourse with a third party. Either of these actions represents a reproductive intervention that raises problems similar to those associated with AID and should be regarded as ethically unacceptable.

In Vitro Fertilisation. *In vitro* fertilisation may be considered in the management of women with absent or severely damaged fallopian tubes; the procedure might also have a place in the management of some cases of infertility due to oligospermia, sperm antibodies, hostile cervical mucus, or even some patients with unexplained infertility. It has been achieved in the human as follows: fluid was aspirated from a pre-ovulatory ovarian follicle and an oocyte recovered from that fluid; the oocyte was then cultured *in vitro* under controlled conditions. Semen was obtained by masturbation and the spermatozoa were separated from the semenal plasma by gentle centrifugation. Fertilisation took place in a culture medium and the embryo was inserted into the uterine cavity about sixty hours after fertilisation.[4] In 1980, Steptoe and colleagues gave details of four pregnancies established by fertilisation *in vitro*, followed by the planting of cleaving embryos into the mothers. These pregnancies were monitored by hormone assays in early pregnancy and by ultrasound scans. Amniocentesis was used to exclude open neural tube defects and to effect a chromosome analysis of the foetus. Three of the pregnancies began uneventfully and the foetuses were normal in all respects; two were delivered at or near term, but the third aborted while the patient was on holidays. The fourth pregnancy did not develop normally and an abnormal foetus was aborted spontaneously twelve weeks after the last menstrual period.

The ethical problems that arise with *in vitro* fertilisation are multiple. They involve considerations of the beginning of human life and the value of life, in addition to the obvious questions of parenthood and sex. The first serious ethical problem that arises with *in vitro* fertilisation is its experimental character. It has been argued that, given the unknown hazard associated with laboratory culture and embryonic transfer and the inability to overcome such unknown hazards, *in vitro* fertilisation with subsequent implantation constitutes potentially hazardous experimentation with a human subject without his consent.

Furthermore, *in vitro* fertilisation raises the immediate question of the risk of deformity though one must also recall that this risk is present when fertilisation occurs in a natural physiological manner. Nonetheless, the development of successful test-tube babies has, to date, been monitored by amniocentesis, no doubt with the intention of terminating a pregnancy if an abnormality were detected. If such management is necessary for the use of *in vitro* fertilisation, the the procedure must be deemed to be ethically unacceptable.

A further and perhaps more important consideration is the question of possible embryo wastage. If multiple fertilisation occurred and only one embyro transferred back into the mother, the remaining embryos would presumably be discarded. People who are convinced that human personhood begins with fertilisation would reject *in vitro* fertilisation on those grounds, for it would involve deliberate destruction of human life to achieve pregnancy.

The Foster Womb. A woman in whom the fertilised egg (other than her own) is implanted is a 'host' mother, who offers her womb as a foster womb. A great variety of situations and motivations can be imagined. A healthy woman might not want to jeopardise or interrupt her career by the inconvenience of a pregnancy. Another might desire a child, but be anguished by the prospect of pregnancy and childbirth. The health of still another might not allow a pregnancy although she wanted a child. All these women might seek a foster mother in whom an embryo would be implanted following *in vitro* fertilisation of the sperm and ovum of the couple who desired the child. The ethical problems that arise are numerous. What if the 'host' mother becomes psychologically attached to that which is physically attached to her? What if the genetic mother who has good intentions at the start of the procedure, finds herself some months later psychologically unable to accept the child who has been carried and borne by another woman? Because of problems such as these, most people would consider the foster womb as always being unethical.[5]

The Artificial Placenta. A foetus, born as early as 24 or 25 weeks after conception may sometimes survive with modern management. Attempts have also been made to keep alive human foetuses expelled by miscarriages as early as 10 weeks after conception. The idea of an artificial placenta raises the possibility of the complete gestation of a child outside the womb, from fertilisation. This laboratory production of human beings has been called by Leon Kass 'the complete dehumanisation of procreation'. Others have called the procedure 'an unethical experimentation with human beings'. Many would hold that, even if the biological risk of such practice could be reduced to normal proportions, the procedure would still be unacceptable, at least because of the grave psychological danger for a foetus bred outside the human milieu, without the essential symbiotic mother/child relationship. Here there would be complete separation of human generation from conjugal love.

The present chapter has summarised the main causes of infertility and given a résumé of the methods of investigating and treating the infertile couple. Infertility can, on occasions, cause grave psychological problems and it is important that every couple is treated with tact and understanding. Some forms of treatment do present ethical problems and the reasons for not using some forms of therapy must be carefully and sympathetically explained to each couple who, after all, are only trying to reproduce their species.

6

Natural Family Planning

JOHN BONNAR

> To everything there is a season, and a time to every
> purpose under the Heaven:
> A time to be born, and a time to die . . .
> A time for making love and a time for not making love.
> (*Ecclesiastes* 3)

Introduction

Natural family planning (NFP) is the term used for fertility regulation based on the observation of the naturally occurring signs and symptoms of the fertile and infertile phases of the menstrual cycle. NFP can be used either to avoid or to achieve pregnancy and is of interest to many millions throughout the world who for religious or cultural reasons do not want to use contraceptive drugs or devices. Dissatisfaction with current contraceptive technology and concern about side-effects and morbidity are other reasons for many turning to NFP. The use of hormones and chemicals for birth control is also being questioned by various groups concerned with ecology and by those who wish to encourage natural childbirth and breast-feeding. Recently, several developed and developing countries (USA, Republic of Ireland, Brazil and Chile) have introduced legislation that NFP methods must be made available in their national family planning programmes.

The current methods of NFP are based on the concept of fertility awareness, namely the woman's ability to identify on a day-to-day basis certain physiological changes which depend on follicular maturation and ovulation; these have largely replaced the so called rhythm methods which depended upon prediction of the fertile times. Natural family planning also includes the birth spacing role of breast feeding; on a world-wide scale lactation is responsible for more fertility control than all the contraceptive methods in current use (Rosa 1976; Short 1976). In contrast to the pill and intrauterine devices which require a medical delivery system, natural family planning involves an educational and learning process not directly involving doctors. When pregnancy is not desired abstinence from intercourse ('days of rest') is an essential component of

NFP and the modification of sexual behaviour which is involved has important psychosexual aspects.

Ogino and Knaus. The application of female reproductive physiology to to the control of fertility based on cyclical sexual activity dates from the independent work of Ogino (1930) in Japan and Knaus (1930) in Austria in the 1930s. Both showed that, independent of the length of the individual cycle, the timing of ovulation is relatively constant in relation to the succeeding menstruation and not to the previous menses. From these studies both developed formulas to determine the fertile and infertile days of the menstrual cycle. The term 'rhythm' came into use following the work of Ogino and Knaus and was used to describe methods of birth control based on the cyclic pattern of fertile and infertile days. Major reviews of this area have been provided by Hartman (1962). Ross and Piotrow (1974), and Vollman (1977).

Methods of Natural Family Planning

Over the last few years the term *natural family planning* has been introduced to describe the various methods of birth control based on fertility awareness and cyclical sexual intercourse. The World Health Organisation (WHO) has recommended the following definition:

> Natural family planning refers to techniques for planning or preventing pregnancies by observation of naturally occurring signs and symptoms of the fertile and infertile phases of the menstrual cycle. It is implicit in the definition of natural family planning when used to avoid pregnancies that there is abstinence from sexual intercourse during the fertile phase of the menstrual cycle. (Lanctot 1979)

The emphasis in current NFP methods is to determine the beginning and the end of the potentially fertile period. A frequent misunderstanding is the assumption that these methods are used to detect the time of ovulation. To date the major methods of NFP can be classified into four categories (i) calculation or calendar method (ii) basal body temperature method (iii) ovulation or cervical mucus method (iv) symptothermal methods.

(i) ***Calculation or calendar method.*** The calculation or calendar method is the oldest technique for determining the fertile period and came into use in the 1930s after the work of Ogino and Knaus. In brief, the calendar method involves identifying the fertile time from the records of the previous 6–12 menstrual cycles. Knaus (1933), maintained that ovulation occurred on the fifteenth day before menstruation whereas Ogino (1930) calculated that ovulation could take place at a variable time between the twelfth and sixteenth days before menstruation. The method allowed seventy-two hours for the survival of sperm capable of fertilising the ovum and the latter a life span of 12–24 hours. The potential fertile period was then calculated on the following basis:

1. Define the shortest and the longest menstrual cycle over the preceding six and preferably twelve cycles.
2. The first day of the potentially fertile period is the shortest cycle minus 18 days.
3. The last day of the potentially fertile period is the longest cycle minus 11 days.

For a woman whose menstrual cycles have varied from 26–31 days, application of the calendar month would mean a potentially fertile period as follows:

First day of potential fertility: 26–18 = 8
Last day of potential fertility: 31–11 = 20

This would mean that she was possibly fertile from the 8–20th day of the cycle.

The greatest weakness of the calendar method is that it depends on a prediction, based on the menstrual history, of what is likely to occur and not on what is actually taking place. While the method is of value to the woman with regular cycles, those with irregular cycles will have prolonged periods of potential fertility which will render the method of low acceptability due to the prolonged abstinence involved. In the age group 20 – 40 years menstrual cycles are much more likely to be regular but can deviate widely in the individual woman (Treloar *et al*. 1967).

(ii) ***Basal Body Temperature Method.*** The temperature or thermal method depends upon the identification of the rise in the basal body temperature (BBT) from a relatively lower level during the follicular phase to a relatively higher level during the luteal phase of the menstrual cycle. This occurs around the time of ovulation due to the thermogenic effect of progesterone. Moghissi, Synar and Evans (1972) found that the BBT rose simultaneously with the luteinising hormone surge and the significant rise in BBT coincided with the rise of plasma progesterone to a mean level of 4 ng/ml and urinary pregnanediol to greater than 1.8 ng/24 hrs. The BBT remained elevated until the progesterone level fell below these concentrations.

The shift in temperature is small, between 0.2–0.5°C (0.4–1.0°F), usually occurs abruptly over 24 hours and is sometimes preceded by a small dip in the temperature. A significant temperature shift is defined as one that occurs in 48 hours or less, and in which three consecutive daily temperatures are at least 0.2°C higher than the last six daily temperatures prior to the start of the shift. The temperature rise associated with ovulation may also be gradual or step-like in pattern over several days.

For an extensive review of the temperature patterns of the menstrual cycle the reader is referred to the work of Marshall (1965), Vollman (1977), Hartman (1962), Zuspan and Zuspan (1979). If fertilisation of the ovum occurs, the temperature remains at the higher level but otherwise it usually falls shortly before or during menstruation. Since it is a shift in BBT rather than the temperature itself which is important the readings need to be taken daily and at the same time. Special 'ovulation' thermometers with expanded scales and charts which facilitate the identification of the temperature shift have been developed. Records of BBT kept on ordinary clinical temperature charts are of little value. Ideally, the temperature should be recorded in the morning on waking after at least 3–5 hours of uninterrupted sleep, before rising from bed, and before eating or drinking. The temperature can be taken in the mouth, axilla vagina or rectum providing the same procedure is always used. More important is the scale of the graph paper or chart used for recording the temperature. A scale where the space covered by two days on the horizontal axis is equal to the space of 0.1°C on the vertical axis facilitates the identification of the shift (Spieler 1980) – see figure 1 on p.72.

The BBT method did not become widely used for family planning until the 1950s. The method is used either alone or in combination with a calendar calculation which determines the beginning of the fertile period. Using the BBT method alone the end of the fertile period is recognised by the sustained elevation of the BBT for three days after the rise, and coitus is confined to the post ovulation and infertile phase of the cycle. A 'coverline' drawn 0.05°C above the highest of the lower follicular phase temperatures and including at least six normal temperatures is used to define the three higher temperatures (figure 1).

A combination of an Ogino-based calculation to identify the onset of the fertile phase and the daily BBT to indicate the end of the fertile phase is more commonly used. The first day of the fertile period is calculated by subtracting 19 days, viz. Ogino-formula plus one day from the shortest known cycle based on the preceding twelve menstrual cycles. If only six consecutive cycles are recorded the first day of the fertile period is calculated by subtracting twenty days from the shortest observed cycle. If the woman has no previous records of her menstrual cycles, up to the sixth day of the cycle can be considered infertile provided the previous cycle was ovulatory as shown by a biphasic temperature chart. Roetzer (1978) reported only one pregnancy from coitus on the sixth day of the cycle in 8,532 cycles in couples using early infertile days.

Women experienced in the BBT method often discontinue temperature readings once the post-ovulation phase is established and do not resume temperature recordings until after menstruation.

Vollman (1977) has made an outstanding contribution to knowledge of the menstrual cycle and analysed BBT recordings of 20,672 cycles in 621 women. In short menstrual cycles (7–17 days) monophasic temperature curves occurred in 57.1 per cent. The incidence of monophasic curves decreased with an increase in length of the menstrual cycles and dropped to 5.8 per cent at cycles of 24 days. In cycles of 25–32 days the incidence of monophasic curves was lowest at 1.8 to 4.8 per cent. With increasing length of the menstrual cycle beyond 32 days the rate of monophasic BBT curves steadily increased, reaching 41.3 per cent in cycles of sixty days and longer. Monophasic charts also showed, as expected, an age-dependent distribution. In the year of the menarche monophasic BBT curves were observed in 55.7 per cent of menstrual cycles and the incidence decreased sharply during adolescence. In mature women the rate of monophasic curves was around 2 per cent, and as low as 1.2 per cent between 23 and 29 years. In the pre-menopausal years the incidence of monophasic cycles rose to 34 per cent.

The use of the BBT method alone or in combination with a calculation for the start of the fertile period may be more acceptable where cycles are regular and short, but will meet with problems in the presence of long and anovulatory cycles. A woman depending on BBT will not know whether the absence of a temperature rise was due to an anovulatory infertile cycle or to a delayed ovulation. Women approaching the menopause, or following childbirth may therefore encounter this difficulty quite frequently. The major drawback of the temperature method alone is the need for abstention from intercourse until the post-ovulation phase as no information is provided about the onset of the fertile period.

(iii) ***Ovulation Method.*** The basis of the ovulation method is that the cervical glands are a highly sensitive target of the oestrogen level in the blood and therefore accurately reflect follicular maturation in the ovary. Billings *et al.* (1972) reported that cervical mucus symptoms appeared at a mean of 6.2 days before ovulation defined as occurring the day after the mid-cycle peak of luteinising hormone. This was confirmed in 1976 by Flynn and Lynch (1976) who investigated hormonal parameters of ovulation and mucus symptoms and found that the mucus first appeared at a mean of 5.3 days before the day of the luteinising hormone peak.

Hilgers, Abraham and Cavanagh (1978) also correlated mucus symptoms with the estimated time of ovulation, which was calculated as the mid-point between the days that the plasma progesterone level reached between 1 ng and 2.3 ng/ml. In sixty-four out of sixty-five cycles the estimated time of ovulation occurred from three days before to three days after the peak symptom – the last day of fertile type mucus. In 95.4 per cent of cycles the estimated time of ovulation occurred within plus or minus 2 days of the 'peak', and the mean number of mucus days preceding ovulation was 5.9 days. The authors considered that the most significant finding of the study was that in 63 out of 65 normal ovulatory cycles (97 per cent) the estimated time of ovulation was during the time of fertility as defined by the ovulation method.

To use the ovulation method, the woman has to learn to recognise the sequence of changes in the quality and quantity of her mucus and the associated sensation at the vulva. For a detailed description of the method the reader is referred to Billings, Billings and Catarinich (1977) and McCarthy, Martin and Gildenhorn (1978) and the Family Fertility Learning Package produced by the World Health Organisation (1979). Women are taught that:

1. Menstrual bleeding is followed by a variable number of 'dry' days when no mucus secretion is present and the genital area feels 'dry' due to the low level of oestrogen.
2. The end of the dry sensation indicates that the production of mucus has started. The type of mucus rather than the quantity is important. Infertile type mucus is opaque and described as tacky, sticky and crumbly and may be white or yellow.
3. The fertile type mucus is slippery and wet with the consistency of raw egg white and may stretch without breaking (spinnbarkeit). The mucus may be clear but is sometimes cloudy or stained with blood and hence brown, yellow, pink or red. Even if no mucus is seen the slippery sensation will indicate its presence. During this phase, oestrogen levels reach their peak and the mucus is highly favourable for sperm transport and survival. The last day of the fertile type mucus is called the 'peak' day and occurs close to the time of ovulation.
4. In the post-ovulation phase the mucus either changes back to the infertile sticky, non-stretchy, non-slippery type, or disappears completely so that there is a definite sensation of dryness. The precise characteristics of the mucus and the length of the different phases vary among individual women.

The ovulation method is summarised in figure 2. Couples are advised to abstain from intercourse (1) during menstruation because of the possible early onset of the fertile period near the end of the menses, (2) on alternate 'dry' days prior to the onset of the fertile period – to minimise the difficulty of recognising the onset of mucus secretion in the presence of seminal fluid – and (3) during the fertile period itself. Intercourse is resumed on the fourth day after the 'peak' day. Other rules apply to the 'early' days before the onset of the fertile period to enable the woman to recognise her basic infertile pattern, and to the use of the method following childbirth, during lactation and in the pre-menopausal years.

The attraction of the ovulation method is its relative simplicity and independence of any gadgetry. The woman is taught to recognize the presence and significance of the different secretions and sensations at the vaginal area and to make her observations throughout the day prior to and after micturition. She can use toilet tissues or her fingers to tell whether the introitus is dry or wet, as shown by whether the tissue slides easily over the genital area. Tissue paper will also show the mucus and the spinnbarkeit can be tested by folding the tissue. The whole observation should take only a few seconds.

(iv) ***Sympto-Thermal Methods***. These methods of natural family planning incorporate several markers of ovarian function in order to define the infertile period with greater accuracy. This approach to avoiding pregnancy was first popularised in Canada in the 1960s but has since been developed primarily as a combination of the cervical mucus method and the shift of the basal body temperature (McCarthy, Martin and Gildenhorn (1978); Parenteau-Carreau, Lanctot and Rice (1976); World Health Organisation (1979). To a lesser extent the woman may also use other symptoms or signs such as mid-cycle pain or bleeding, breast fullness or tenderness, and changes of the cervix (figure 1). Self observation of changes in the cervix were first reported by Keefe (1962) and the correlation with ovarian function has been well demonstrated by Insler *et al.* (1972) and Flynn (1973).

The rules of the sympto-thermal methods are as follows:

1. the first day of the fertile period is determined by (*a*) the appearance of the cervical mucus and the sensation of 'wetness' in the genital area or (*b*) the shortest cycle of the last 6 minus 20 or minus 19 if records of twelve cycles are available, or (*c*) a combination of both using the earliest reading as the most reliable.
2. the onset of the post-ovulatory infertile phase is determined by (*a*) the day of the third high temperature after the rise if the mucus has disappeared or has lost its fertile characteristics, or (*b*) the fourth day after the 'peak' mucus symptom, whichever is the latest.

For full details of the instruction required in sympto-thermal methods the reader is referred to the manuals published by the Human Life and Natural Family Planning Foundation (McCarthy *et al.* 1978) and to the Family Fertility Education Package of the World Health Organisation (1979). As in the ovulation method, the woman in special circumstances such as after childbirth, breast-feeding or approaching the menopause requires instruction in additional refinements of the method.

International Studies on Natural Family Planning

In 1977 the World Health Organisation set up a multi-centre study to determine the percentage of women capable of recognising the changes in the cervical mucus during the menstrual cycle and the use-effectiveness of this approach to family planning. Women were recruited from five countries, namely El Salvador, India, Ireland, New Zealand and the Philippines. All were of proven fertility with no previous training in natural family planning, representative of various cultures and socio-economic levels and ranging in educational status from illiteracy to postgraduate education. The results of the study have recently been reported (World Health Organisation 1981). The most striking finding of the teaching phase was that in the first cycle following instruction 93 per cent of the women were able to recognise and record their mucus symptoms, which allowed self-recognition of the fertile period. A previous study in British women who were instructed by correspondence showed that 75 per cent of the subjects observed mucus symptoms in every cycle (Marshall 1975). In the WHO study self-recognition of cervical mucus was achieved regardless of the educational level; 94 per cent of women in El Salvador produced an interpretable mucus pattern although 92.5 per cent had less than six years schooling and 47.8 per cent were illiterate. The subject's understanding of the method was assessed as 'excellent' or 'good' in 91 per cent after the first cycle, increasing to 94 per cent and 97 per cent after the second and third cycles. The WHO study tends to suggest that women of low socio-economic status and education in developing countries can learn the self-recognition of the fertile period by the mucus symptoms more readily than highly educated women in developed countries. Another surprising finding was that a history of vaginal discharge did not affect the ability of the woman to recognise the mucus symptoms. A total of 5.2 per cent of the 870 women who entered the teaching phase became pregnant, the rate being highest in El Salvador (8 per cent) and lowest in Ireland (3 per cent); these were classified mainly as due to 'conscious departure from the rules of the method' or inaccurate application of the instructions. Another important finding of the study was that the pregnancy rate was highest in those women who required teaching for more than three cycles; those learning the method within three cycles had 1.3 pregnancies per cycle and those requiring extended teaching beyond three cycles had 7.02 per cent pregnancies per cycle. The discontinuation rate in the teaching phase of the WHO study was low and 85 per cent of the women entered the effectiveness phase. In a recent study of the ovulation method in North America the continuation rate at three months was 77 per cent with a 6.5 per cent pregnancy rate (Wade *et al.* 1979).

Effectiveness of Natural Family Planning

Considerable reservations have been felt about many of the older studies on NFP methods as they were usually retrospective and lacking in information on selection, discontinuations and follow-up. More recently, the scientific methodology developed by Tietze (1962) for field trials of contraceptives has been applied to NFP. Marshall (1968) was among the first to carry out a prospective field trial of the temperature method. Several of the major prospective studies in NFP are summarised in table 1 (p.71) which gives the pregnancy rates in terms of method failure (theoretical effectiveness) and of combined method and user effectiveness. The pearl formula or number of pregnancies per hundred women years of exposure is used for comparison, as the more precise life table form of analysis is only available for the most recent studies.

Using the BBT method alone for family planning, Marshall (1968) in a study of 321 women over 4,749 cycles with coitus confined to the post-ovulatory infertile phase obtained a method failure of 1.2 pregnancies per 100 women years. If a combination of calculation and BBT was used with coitus in both the pre and post-ovulatory infertile phases, Marshall (1968) found the method failure rate was 5 pregnancies per 100 women years. Doring (1973) in a retrospective study of 11,352 cycles reported only one pregnancy (0.11 pregnancies per 100 women years) due to a false interpretation of the temperatures because of a head cold and 8 pregnancies in all, which he considered the result of errors on the part of the users.

Weissmann *et al.* (1972) reported on the first prospective study of the ovulation method in 282 women in the Pacific Island of Tonga over a total of 2503 months. From the start of instruction to the conclusion, 81 women became pregnant but of these, 28 abandoned the method, 50 ignored the indication of possible fertility, 2 conceived because of error in the application of the rules and only one was classified as a method failure. The study of Ball (1976) of the ovulation method in Australia reported a method failure rate of 2.9 pregnancies per 100 women years and a user failure rate of 12.5 pregnancies per 100 women years. Two recent studies of the ovulation method in North America have been reported. Wade *et al.* (1979) undertook a randomised prospective study to compare the ovulation method with the sympto-thermal method. In 404 couples assigned to the ovulation method the discontinuation rate due to pregnancy was 22.9 per cent in the first year from the start of the training period. Klauss *et al.* (1979) in a six-centre study reported on 1,139 subjects followed up to 24 months (12,283 cycles). Method failure rates at 12 and 24 months for the ovulation group was 1.29 and 1.17 pregnancies per 100 women years. Combined method and user failure rates were approximately 20 pregnancies per 100 women years.

The first international multi-centre evaluation of effectiveness of the ovulation method was carried out by the World Health Organisation (1981). Combining the data from the teaching phase and effectiveness phases, a total of 20 per cent of the 870 subjects admitted to the study became pregnant: 45 of the 870 subjects (5.2 per cent) during the teaching phase and 129 of 708 (18 per cent) during the effectiveness phase. Using life table analysis for the effectiveness phase the overall net cumulative rate of discontinuation because of pregnancy was 20 per cent ranging from 14 per cent in the Philippines to 28 per cent in New Zealand. The method failure rates for the effectiveness study ranged from 2.1 to 3.7 and except for New Zealand the method was shown to be theoretically 97–99 per cent effective. The main reason for pregnancy during the study was the decision by the couple not to abstain during the fertile period. This contributed to more than two-thirds of the pregnancies – 15.6 pregnancies per 100 women years. Inaccurate application of the instructions was responsible for 3.8 pregnancies per 100 women years. The continuation rate for the whole study was 56.2 per cent at 16 cycles.

Couples who follow the rules of NFP methods have without doubt effective methods of fertility regulation with method failure rates of 0.5 – 3.0 pregnancies per 1,300 cycles but in general use the methods are around 80 per cent effective. The continuation rate for the NFP methods compares favourably with intrauterine devices and oral contraceptives. Intrauterine devices are estimated to have a net pregnancy rate of 1–6 per cent at the end of the first year after insertion and in a recent WHO study of intrauterine devices in current use continuation rates at 12 and 24 months ranged from 54–61 per cent and 43–51 per cent respectively (World Health Organisation 1980). Oral contraception has a failure rate of approximately 1 per 100 women years but the net probability of discontinuation at one year is around 50 per cent. In unreliable tablet takers the cumulative probability of pregnancy reaches 8.3 per cent at one year for combined oral contraception and 13.4 per cent for low-dose progestogen only pills. Discontinuation for the latter reached 61 per cent at 12 months and 76 per cent at 22 months.

Few studies have been undertaken to compare acceptability and effectiveness of the ovulation method and the sympto-thermal method. A random allocation of these two methods was undertaken by Wade *et al.* (1979) in California. The pregnancy rate was 24.8 per cent among ovulation method users and 9.4 per cent for sympto-thermal users. These differences were significant indicating a higher acceptance and effectiveness rate for the sympto-thermal method in the population studied. In contrast, a WHO study (Medina and Cifuentes, 1979) in Columbia found no significant difference in the 12-month pregnancy rates for the ovulation method (19 per cent) and the sympto-thermal method (22 per cent).

Johnston, Roberts and Spencer (1978) reported an extensive study in Australian couples using three varieties of NFP: sympto-thermal with a calendar calculator to determine the beginning of the fertile period, sympto-thermal using the mucus signs to determine the onset of the fertile period and the ovulation method itself. The overall pregnancy rates were 8.6, 15.9 and 27.6 per cent pregnancies per 100 women years. The authors acknowledge that the different NFP methods did not have the same teaching or follow-up. The analysis has been criticised as being more retrospective than prospective but it provides a wealth of data on acceptance rates, discontinuation and the problems of delivery of NFP in the context of a poor distribution of NFP services in competion with readily available contraceptive methods. Johnston *et al.* (1978) suggests that important factors influencing continuity/discontinuation include the NFP method learned, the place where the client learns the method, the experience which the client accumulates on the method and the ability of the couple to modify the frequency of intercourse.

Breast-Feeding and Birth Spacing

In western societies, it is a common belief among pregnant women, doctors and nurses that a large number of women are now physiologically incapable of breast-feeding. For the great majority of babies throughout the world successful lactation by the mother is a sine qua non of survival. In the space of a few generations the efficiency of lactation for many women in the developed countries has been compromised and for some, breast-feeding has become impossible. Short (1976) suggests that the over-emphasis of the breast as a sexual symbol may have caused cultural imprinting which makes it difficult for the woman to come to terms with breast-feeding and she feels ashamed to suckle her child in case it is interpreted as an obscene act.

Breast-feeding has been the key physiological mechanism of birth spacing and the decline of this natural control of fertility has been largely responsible for the recent exponential increase in the world's population (Short 1976). Research in developing countries has shown the profound effect of breast-feeding on fertility (Van Ginneken 1977). Among the Kung hunter gatherers of the Kalahari breast-feeding without supplementation continues for 3–4 years and this results in an average birth interval of 35.4 months. A recent study of the nursing frequency, gonadal function and birth spacing indicates that the pattern of brief and frequent nursing is apparently responsible for the suppression of ovulation (Konner and Worthman 1980). Kung infants sleep with their mothers until weaned and also breast-feed at night without waking the mother. In Rwanda, rural women breast-feed on demand and 50 per cent conceive again within 23 months after delivery; in urban women, breast-feeding follows a more rigid schedule with fewer feeding episodes and 50 per cent conceive again within 9 months of delivery (Howie and McNeilly 1979). This evidence suggests that the patterns of frequent suckling without supplementation play an important role in maintaining the birth spacing effect of prolonged lactation.

The role of lactation in the regulation of fertility has been disregarded in western societies on the grounds that it is unreliable. The duration of lactational amenorrhoea in women is variable but full lactation delays menstruation longer than partial lactation (Perez *et al.* 1972; Rosa 1976). Suckling leads to the release of prolactin from the anterior pituitary, and in prolonged lactation basal prolactin levels are related both to the frequency of suckling and to the duration of lactational amenorrhoea (Gross and Eastman 1979; Howie and McNeilly 1979). The data of Gross and

Eastman (1979) also suggests that in prolonged lactation an elevated prolactin level continues to exert an effect on ovarian function without necessarily producing amenorrhoea.

During pregnancy the level of follicle stimulating hormone (FSH) is suppressed by the high levels of oestrogen but after delivery the level of FSH reaches the normal follicular range by 15–20 days postpartum (Bonnar *et al.* 1975). Bonnar *et al.* found that in non-lactating women oestradiol levels began to rise by day 17 postpartum when the level of prolactin had returned to normal, indicating the return of follicular activity. In contrast, oestradiol levels remain suppressed in lactating women indicating an absence of follicular development in the ovary despite normal FSH levels. It is uncertain whether prolactin acts directly on the ovary or the hypothalamus or both (Howie and McNeilly 1979). The mechanism of lactational amenorrhoea is still poorly understood. It would seem that the raised prolactin levels induced by suckling inhibit the normal positive feedback effect of oestrogen on the hypothalamus. As a result, production of LH Releasing Hormone is diminished and ovulation is prevented through the loss of pulsatile secretion of LH from the pituitary (Howie and McNeilly 1979).

From the viewpoint of fertility control, it should be recognised that traditional breast-feeding has a central regulating role in the spacing of births and is of immense importance where methods of fertility control are either not acceptable or not available. The introduction of infant feeding programmes which change traditional practices of breast-feeding will therefore interfere with the physiological mechanisms whereby lactation inhibits reproduction. There is also general agreement that oestrogen containing contraceptives have an adverse effect on lactation (Thomson, Hytten and Black 1975).

As yet, no large prospective studies of the use of NFP methods in breast-feeding mothers have been reported. The use of the ovulation method and sympto-thermal methods during breast-feeding are described in several NFP publications (Billings, Billings and Caterinich 1977; McCarthy, Martin and Gildenhorn 1978). A detailed description of the use of the ovulation method during breast-feeding for African women in Nigeria has been provided by McSweeney (1979). The postpartum period is a major area for research in family planning and the use of NFP methods to detect returning fertility in both lactating and non-lactating mothers needs to be evaluated.

Psychosocial and Psychosexual Aspects of Natural Family Planning

The psychosocial and psychosexual aspects of all methods of fertility control are areas of major importance where very little research has been carried out. Couples' decisions regarding the number and spacing of births are influenced by a wide range of cultural, socio-economic and psychological factors. With the exception of a few reports (Marshall and Rowe 1972) virtually no behavioural science studies have been attempted in the area of NFP. The need for research in this area is highlighted by the fact that couples knowingly 'taking a chance' during the fertile period are responsible for a high proportion of the unplanned pregnancies. Although problems exist with the delivery and continuation of all fertility regulation methods, certain areas are unique to NFP. These include the couple involvement, identification of the fertile and infertile days, the change of sexual behaviour and implementation of abstinence if pregnancy is not desired.

Several areas identified by the World Health Organisation which are in need of research include:

(i) factors influencing demand, choice and use of NFP methods. Studies which show comparison with other methods of fertility control are required.
(ii) the effects of fertility regulating methods on family dynamics and marital harmony and their impact on conjugal stability.
(iii) the psychosocial characteristics related to success or failure with NFP.
(iv) the modes of presentation of NFP which stimulate demand, increase acceptance and promote compliance with the requirements of NFP methods.

It is hoped that objective research in these areas can be pursued in the near future. Initially research may need to be directed to finding the ways in which valid information can be obtained about various aspects of human sexual behaviour, attitudes to fertility regulation and the factors influencing motivation and compliance. The whole area is certainly worthy of the attention of social and behavioural scientists.

Research and Development of New Methods to Determine the Fertile Period

Easy to use and inexpensive tests to identify the fertile period and ovulation would be useful for fertility control. Such technology would also find immediate application for the diagnosis and therapy of infertility. At present, a thermometer is the only device available for home use which enables women to detect ovulation, and simple chemical tests or kits for predicting ovulation are not available. The self-observation of the changes of cervical mucus is the only method to identify the fertile period.

The WHO Task Force on Methods for Determination of the Fertile Period is currently working on the development of new technology in this field (Spieler 1980). Research supported by the Task Force has shown that unitary metabolites of oestrogen (estrone – 3 – glucuronide) and progesterone (pregnanediol – 3 – glucuronide) may provide the basis of kits for the prediction and detection of ovulation. The development of simple non-isotopic methods for the *detection* of ovulation which will replace current laboratory methods seems highly feasible. The adaptation of such methods into kits for do-it-yourself home use is a likely possibility. Kits for the *prediction* of ovulation based on oestrogen glucuronides require much greater sensitivity and precision and are likely to be more difficult although still feasible.

Many attempts have been made to develop devices other than the BBT thermometer to detect ovulation. Claims have been made that ovulation can be detected by devices for home use which measure electro or biopotential differences. Independent studies of such instruments have so far shown them to be unreliable and of no value for identifying the fertile period or the time of ovulation (Bonnar 1977). Electronic thermometers are now available and the technology exists to incorporate programmes which would store the temperatures and detect the shift of the BBT. This would facilitate the detection of ovulation and the identification of the post-ovulatory infertile phase of the menstrual cycle. Devices for field testing this approach will soon be available (World Health Organisation 1980).

Conclusion

The existence of the fertile and infertile phases of the menstrual cycle is now established and natural methods of family planning are now available based on the self-recognition of the fertile phase. Couples who follow the rules of NFP methods have highly effective methods of fertility regulation with method failure rates of 0.5 to 3.0 pregnancies in 1,300 cycles but in general use, the methods are around 80 per cent effective. Continuation rates for NFP compare favourably with intra-uterine devices and oral contraception.

The major advantage of natural family planning is that no hormones or chemicals are introduced into the woman's body. The method is couple orientated and promotes self-knowledge and autonomy. NFP requires an educational approach rather than a medical delivery system and aims to make the users both autonomous and potential educators of other users. The major problem with NFP is the modification of sexual behaviour which is involved and the high degree of motivation required for successful use. Women of low socio-economic or educational level would seem to be able to learn and use the methods more easily than highly educated women. Kits for home use which will predict and identify ovulation may soon be available but it remains to be seen whether these will increase acceptability or improve user-effectiveness of NFP.

SELECT BIBLIOGRAPHY

Baillargeon, J., Pelletier-Baillargeon, H. (1963): 'La regulation des naissances', Montreal: *Les Editions du Jour*, 159.

Ball, M. (1976): 'A prospective field trial of the ovulation method of avoiding conception', *Europ. J. Obstet. Gynec. Reprod. Biol.*, 6: 63–6.

Billings, E.L., Billings, J.J. and Catarinich, M. (1977): *Atlas of the Ovulation Method* 3rd ed., Melbourne: Advocate Press.

Billings, E.L., Billings, J.J., Brown, J.B. and Burger, H.G. (1972): Symptoms and hormonal changes accompanying ovulation', *Lancet*, 1, 282–4.

Bonnar, J., Franklin, M., Nott, P.N. and McNeilly, A.S. (1975): 'Effect of breast-feeding on pituitary-ovarian function after childbirth', *Br. Med. J.*, IV, 82–4.

Bonnar, J. (1977): *Report to the World Health Organisation (Special Programme for Research in Human Reproduction) on detection of ovulation in the human by measurement of skin biopotential changes.*

Doring, G.K. (1973): 'Detection of ovulation by the basal body temperature method', in *Proceedings of a Research Conference on Natural Family Planning*, edited by W.A. Uricchio and M.K. Williams, Washington, D.C.: The Human Life Foundation, 171–80.

Flynn, A.M., and Bertrand, P.V. (1973): 'The valve of a cervical score in the assessment of ovarian function in women', *J. Obstet. Gynaec. Br. Cmth.*, 82: 152.

Flynn, A.M., and Lynch, S.S. (1976): 'Cervical mucus and identification of the fertile phase of the menstrual cycle', *Brit. J. Obstet. Gynae.*, 83: 656-9.

Gross, B.A., and Eastman, C.J. (1979): 'Prolactin secretion during prolonged lactational amenorrhoea', *Aust. N.Z. J. Obstet. Gynaec.*, 19: 95–9.

Hartman, C.G. (1962) in: *Science and the Safe Period; a Compendium of Human Reproduction*, Baltimore, Maryland: Williams and Wilkins, 294.

Hilgers, T.W., Abraham, G.E., and Cavanagh, D. (1978): 'Natural family planning: The peak symptom and estimated time of ovulation', *Obstet. Gynec.*, 52: 575.

Howie, P.W., and McNeilly, A.S. (1979): 'Lactational amenorrhoea, prolactin and contraception', *Eur. J. Cl. Investg.*, 9 (4): 237–8.

Insler, V., Melmed, H., Eichenbrenner, I., Serr, D.M., and Lunenfeld, B. (1972): 'The cervical score: a simple semiquantitative method for monitoring of the menstrual cycle', *Int. J. Gynec. Obstet.*, 10 (6): 223–8.

Piotrow, P.T., Rinehart, W., and Schmidt, J.C. (1979): 'Intrauterine Devices', *Population Reports, Series B*, 3.

Johnston, J.A., Roberts, D.B. and Spencer, R.B. (1978): 'A survey evaluation of the efficacy and efficiency of natural family planning services and methods in Australia', *Report of research project*, St. Vincent's Hospital, Sydney, 436.

Keefe, E.P. (1962): Self-observation of the cervix to distinguish days of possible fertility, *Bulletin of the Sloan Hospital for Women*, 8 (4): 129–36.

Klaus, H., Goebel, J.M., Muraski, B., Egizio, M.T., Weitzel, D., Taylor, R.S., Fagan, M.U., Ek, K., and Hobday, K. (1979): 'Use-effectiveness and client satisfaction in six centres teaching the Billings ovulation method', *Contraception*, 19: 613–29.

Knaus, H. (1933): 'Die periodische Frucht- und Unfruchtbarkeit des Weibes', *Zentralblatt für Gynäkologie*, 57 (24), 1393.

Konner, M., and Worthman, C. (1980): 'Nursing frequency, gonadal function, and birth spacing among Kung hunter gatherers', *Science*, 207: 788–91.

Lanctot, C.A. (1979): 'Natural Family Planning', in: *Clinics in Obstetrics and Gynaecology*, 6/I, 109–27, Philadelphia: W.B. Saunders.

Marshall, J. (1965): *Planning for a Family: an atlas of temperature charts*, 159, London: Faber and Faber.

Marshall, J. (1968): 'A field trial of the basal-body temperature method of regulating births', *Lancet*, 2: 8–10.

Marshall, J. (1975): 'The prevalence of mucus discharge as a symptom of ovulation', *J. Biosoc. Sci.*, 7: 49–55.

Marshall, J., and Rowe, B. (1972): 'The effect of personal factors on the use of the basal-body temperature method of regulating birth', *Fert. Steril.*, 23: 417.

McCarthy, J.J., Martin, M.C., and Gildenhorn, M. (1978): *Natural family planning; instructional series for learners*, Washington, D.C.: The Human Life and Natural Family Planning Foundation.

McSweeney, L. (1979): *Love and Life. A guide to birth regulation*, Ibadan, Nigeria: The Caxton Press.

Medina, J.E., and Cifuentes, A. (1979): 'Comparative evaluation of two methods of natural family planning in Columbia', IXth World Congress of Gynaecology and Obstetrics, Tokyo.

Moghissi, K.S., Synar, F.N. and Evans, T.N. (1972): 'A composite picture of the menstrual cycle', *Am. J. Obstet. Gynecol.*, 144: 405.

Ogino, K. (1930): 'Ovulationstermin und Konzeptionstermin'. Zentralblatt für Gynäkologie, 54 (8), 464–79.

Parenteau-Carreau, S., Lanctot, C.A., and Rice, F.J. (1976): 'Etude internationale Fairfield sur l'efficite de la methode sympto-thermique de regulation des naissances. Resultats Canadiens compares aux resultats globaux', *La Vie Medicale au Canada Francais*, 4: 145–53.

Perez, A., Vela, P., Masmick, G.S., and Potter, R.G. (1972): 'First ovulation after childbirth: the effect of breast-feeding', *Am. J. Obstet. Gynecol.*, 114: 1041–7.

Rice, F.J., Lanctot, C.A., and Garcia-Devesa, C. (1977): 'Effectiveness of the sympto-thermal method of natural family planning', presented at the *First General Assembly of the International Federation of Family Life Promotion*, 22–29 June, 1977, California.

Rice, F.J. (1979): 'The Fairfield international collaborative study of the sympto-thermal method', presented at the *Research Workshop on Natural Family Planning*, 27–29 June, 1979, Bethesda.

Roetzer, J. (1978): 'The sympto-thermal method: ten years of change', *Linacre Quarterly*, 45 (4), 358–74.

Rosa, F. (1976): 'Breast-feeding a motive for family planning', *People*, 3: 10–13.

Ross, C., and Piotrow, P.T. (1974): 'Period abstinence: birth control without contraceptives', *Population Report Series I*, No. 1, Washington, D.C.: George Washington University Medical Center, Population Information Programme, 20.

Short, R.V. (1976): 'Lactation – the central control of reproduction in breast-feeding and the mother', *CIBE Foundation Symposium* 45 (new series), Elsevier/North-Holland.

Spieler, J.M. (1980): 'Self-detection of ovulation and the fertile period', *Proceedings of 10th International Congress on Fertility and Sterility, Madrid*, Lancaster: MTP.

Thomson, A.M., Hytten, F.E., and Black, A.E. (1975): 'Lactation and Reproduction', *Bull, World Health Organisation*, 52: 337–49.

Tietze, B. (1962): 'The use effectiveness of contraceptive methods', in: *Research in Family Planning*, edited by C.V. Kaiser, Princeton University Press, 357–69.

Treloar, A.E., Boynton, R.E., Behn, B.G. and Brown, B.W. (1967): 'Variation of the human menstrual cycle through reproductive life', *Int. J. of Fertil.* 12 (I): 77–126.

Van Ginneken, J.K. (1977): 'The chance of contraception during lactation', *J. Biosoc. Sci.* Suppl. 4: 41–54.

Vollman, R.F. (1977): *The Menstrual Cycle*, Philadelphia, W.B. Saunders.

Wade, M.E., McCarthy, P., Abernathy, J.R., Harris, G.S., Danzer, H.C., Uricchio, W.A. (1979): 'A randomised prospective study of the use-effectiveness of two methods of natural family planning: an interim report', *Am. J. Obstet. Gynecol.*, 134: 628–31.

Weissmann, M.C., Foliaki, L., Billings, E.L. and Billings, J.J. (1972): 'A trial of the ovulation method of family planning in Tonga', *Lancet*, ii: 813.

World Health Organisation (1980): *Ninth Annual Report, Special Programme of Research, Development and Research Training in Human Reproduction*, Geneva: WHO, especially 47–59.

World Health Organisation (1980): 'Task Force on Oral Contraceptives. A randomised, double-blind study of two combined oral contraceptives containing the same progestogen but different oestrogens', *Contraception*, 21: 445–59.

World Health Organisation (1979): *Eighth Annual Report, Special Programme of Research, Development and Research Training in Human Reproduction*, Geneva: WHO.

World Health Organisation (1980): Ninth Annual Report, Special Programme of Research, Development and Research Training in Human Reproduction, Geneva: WHO.

World Health Organisation (1981): 'Task Force on Methods for the Determination of the Fertile Period, Special Programme of Research, Development and Research Training in Human Reproduction. A prospective multi-centre trial of the ovulation method of natural family planning: 1 The Teaching Phase' (submitted for publication to the *Am. J. of Obstet. Gynec.*).

World Health Organisation (1981): 'Task Force on Methods for the Determination of the Fertile Period, Special Programme of Research, Development and Research Training in Human Reproduction. A prospective multi-centre trial of the ovulation method of natural family planning: 2. Effectiveness Phase' (submitted to *Brit. J. of Obstet. Gynaec*) 1981.

Zuspan, K.J. and Zuspan, F.P. (1979): 'Basal body temperature', in: *Human Ovulation*, edited by E.S.E. Hafex, Amsterdam, North-Holland, 291–8.

LIFE TABLE ANALYSIS

Comparative Analysis of Effectiveness of Natural Family Planning Methods based on Prospective Studies (1968–1980)

Authors	Year	Method	Subjects	Months	Failure Rate (Pearl Formula) Pregnancies per 100 woman-years	
					Method Related	Combined Methods/ User Failure
Marshall	1968	BBT (post ovulation)	321	4,739	1.2	6.6
Marshall	1968	BBT + calendar calculation (pre & post)	255	3,545	5.0	19.3
Doring	1973	BBT (post ovulation)	307	11,352	0.11	7.0
Weissman	1972	ovulation method (pre & post)	282	2,503	0.48	25.4
Ball	1976	ovulation method (pre & post)	124	1,635	2.9	15.5
Parenteau-Carreau Lanctot & Rice	1976	sympto-thermal (pre & post)	168	3,548	0.7	6.0
Rice, Lanctot & Garcia-Devesa	1979	sympto-thermal (pre & post)	1,022	20,573	0.75	7.5
Wade *et al.*	1979	ovulation method (pre & post)	404	–	–	24.8
Wade *et al.*	1979	sympto-thermal (pre & post)	434	–	–	9.4
Klaus *et al.*	1979	sympto-thermal	1,139	12,283	1.29	20.0
World Health Organisation	1981	ovulation method	870	10,218	2.2	22.4

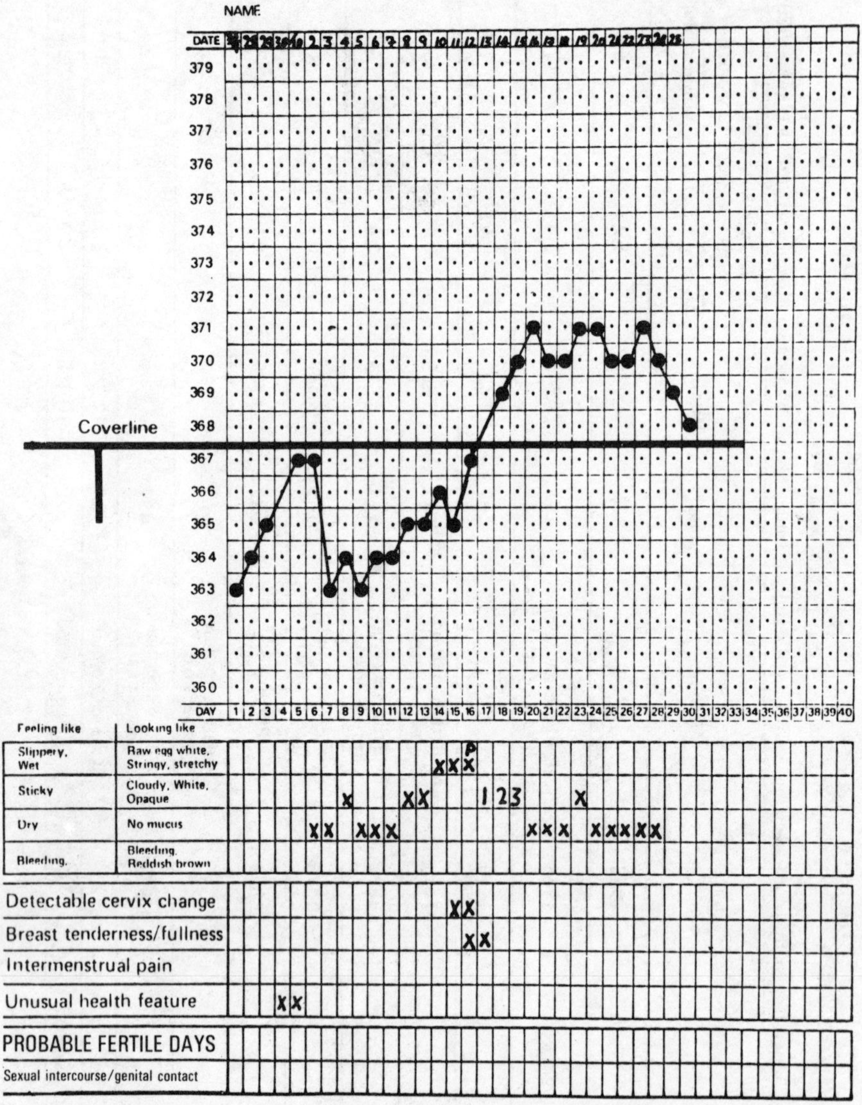

Figure 1. Sympto-Thermal Chart produced by the World Health Organisation (Special Programme for Research in Human Reproduction). The scale of the Temperature Chart facilitates the detection of the temperature shift during the menstrual cycle.

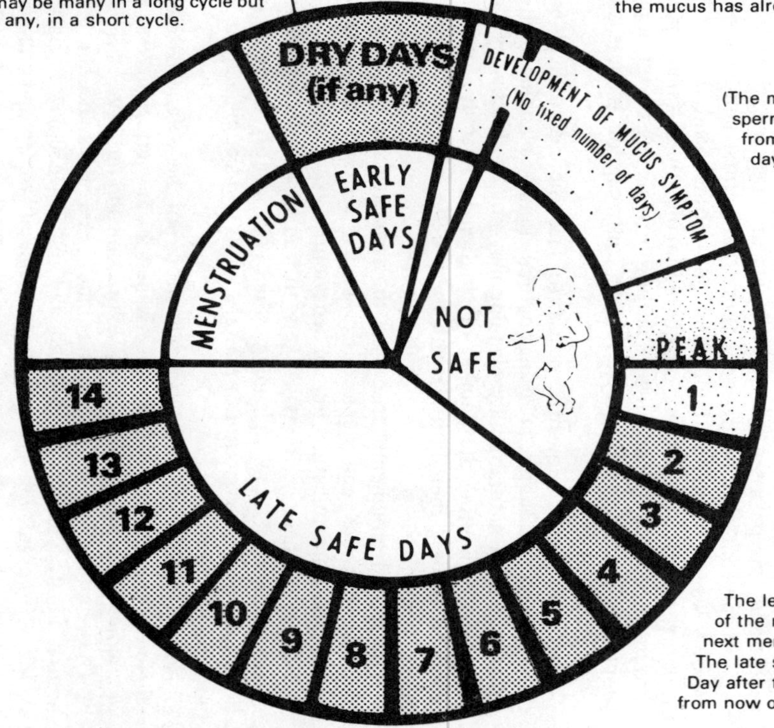

Figure 2. The Ovulation Method which uses the cervical mucus patterns of fertility and infertility.

7

Natural Family Planning: Personal Aspects

DOROTHY SCALLY

Natural family planning has become a very emotive issue, resulting from people adopting polarised stances on it. On the one hand, there are those who, mainly on religious grounds, assert that natural family planning is the only way of planning a family and, on the other hand, there are those who are closed to a serious consideration of natural family planning because they react against religious authority impinging on this aspect of people's behaviour and they believe that contraception is the answer to fertility control.

The first group frequently refuse to face the real difficulties that couples may encounter in using natural family planning and those situations where natural family planning may not be effective as a means of spacing or limiting the number of children in a family, for whatever reason, defending their attitude with the pro-life, pro-baby dimension of their conviction.

The second group emphasise what they perceive as the ineffectiveness of these methods and deplore the sexual restraint they impose as inappropriate and unnatural human behaviour.

Neither of these positions is likely to lead to an objective assessment of any method of family planning, which will identify its strengths and limitations and the conditions necessary for its application and integration into couples' lives.

Natural family planning methods need not be defended solely on religious grounds but on their effectiveness in answering the true needs of couples in relation to their sexual expression and fertility.

These reflections are based on nine years experience in teaching natural family planning to engaged and married couples. In particular, it draws from and builds on the experience of women and couples who have come to a natural family planning centre run, for the past three years, on a one night a week basis. The teachers at this centre are married women and the approach used with our clients is a counselling approach that sees the management of fertility as one aspect of the total marriage relationship and, particularly, of the sexual dimension of that relationship.

I stress this because we have found that no matter how effective a method of family planning is and regardless of how well a woman or a couple understand it, its successful application in their marriage depends largely on the quality of the interpersonal relationship and on factors not directly linked with fertility itself.

Fertility

The first realisation in teaching natural family planning is the degree of ignorance that exists among couples about fertility. Hardly a night at the centre passes without meeting at least one woman who believes she is fertile right through her cycle or has some such misapprehension. Many clients, even though they have conceived, carried and given birth to several babies, have very little knowledge about the process of conception and the development of the fertilised ovum. For this reason, very often, our initial task in fertility guidance is one of giving accurate information about these very processes. The response can be extremely rewarding. It is instructive to see the light of understanding dawn on clients' faces as they learn about this aspect of themselves, realise that there is an actual pattern to their fertility that they can identify, and to watch them reach out to explore the possibilities this raises for them in approaching a management of it. One of the arguments used against natural family planning is that it is complicated and difficult for couples to learn. The question is implicit: why burden couples with the task of recognising and recording their signs of fertility and infertility when a simpler method can be used. Concern in this respect, particularly where more educationally or socially deprived couples are involved, can lead to a judgment against offering them the choice of exploring the possibilities natural family planning methods might hold for them. It is my experience that, generally speaking, people like to know who they are, what they are and why they are; that they value anything they can learn about themselves and believe themselves to be more valuable through the acquiring of such knowledge. In other words, a person's self-esteem and self-respect can grow through self-understanding. When it comes to such an integral and personal aspect as fertility, the acquiring of self-knowledge and awareness is much more likely to be experienced as benefit rather than burden.

The second realisation is that successful family planning is intimately linked with and dependent on the attitudes and approach couples have to intercourse. In fact, I have come to the conclusion that to help with the procreative element of intercourse, one must approach it through the unitive element, if one is to help couples to a wholeness in their sexual experience.

There has been a tendency to abstract the procreative dimension from its context and to treat it in isolation. In the past, procreation has been viewed as the main purpose of intercourse. The pleasure and joy and goodness of the experience was seen as a by-product, as it were, of an act, the function of which was the producing of new life. In more recent times, our understanding of intercourse has changed, and it is realised that the unitive dimension is vital for the continuing growth in love and relationship in marriage. However, instead of leading to a deeper exploration and understanding of the personal meaning of intercourse and the part the procreative dimension plays in it, we have tended to view fertility as a 'problem', attempting to 'treat' it on its own and, thereby, I believe, missing the point altogether. By so doing, it is possible, perhaps, to prevent a pregnancy but also probable to miss out on helping the whole sexual dimension which, I believe, is what good family planning is about. Couples coming to us are certainly seeking a method of avoiding pregnancy, but they are seeking a method which will enable them to experience good sex.

I propose now to look at what is good sex; to look at intercourse as I believe it is meant to be. What follows may seem very idealistic; but, first of all, we must try to define what the ideal is in order to understand the potential and actual experience of couples, and how it affects their attitudes to themselves, to one another and to their fertility. (e.g. Medicine always appeals to the ideal when it refers to the concept of health.)

It could be claimed that intercourse is seldom experienced by many couples in the way I describe it. Yet the ideal as outlined is not alien to the desire and intuition of the couples who visit our centre. It is their expression of what they perceive as good, desirable, whole, as well as their pain in the face of emotional deprivation and the wounds inflicted by meaningless acts that gives shape to the ideal. At the heart of each couple, there is a hunger and need for the experience of the profound personal statement and mutual exchange that the ideal represents and symbolises. The achievement of the ideal may be partial or limited but the recognition of the potential for being truly 'two in one flesh' validates the search and the goal.

Man and woman are drawn to one another, in love, to become one. We seek to find ourselves by giving ourselves. In a sense, we are incomplete until we have found the other, have given ourselves to the other and been received by him or her. Intercourse is one of the most profound ways of expressing this need and of reaching fulfilment. This I believe to be a truth which yet does not deny that other truth – that even in our finding, our giving and receiving, the ultimate fulfilling of our desire lies in eternity. Ideally, when husband and wife have intercourse, it is the ultimate physical expression of two persons acting and interacting together in a shared life that is founded on the love they have for one another.

Intercourse is meant to be an affirmation of the body. Husband and wife look on one another's bodies and find them good. They are drawn to touch, to admire, to desire. It is a very affirming experience to be delighted in at the level of one's body, especially when that delight springs

Erratum: The top three lines of page 77 should read:

from the love and affection for the whole person one is. Intercourse is meant to be joyful and pleasurable; a way of communicating in our flesh what we feel in our hearts.

sexual tension although both of these are good and desirable; it is meant to be a statement about the care and concern we feel for one another at all levels of our daily existence. It is meant to be an expression of our commitment and fidelity to one another; of the way we hold each other. Symbolically we come to intercourse naked, bringing nothing except ourselves in complete intimacy.

Intercourse is meant to be disciplined and responsible. Disciplined, in the sense that the context and environment should be appropriate for its expression. Responsible, in the sense that its consequences should be appreciated and integrated in decisions or choices related to it.

Above all, intercourse is meant to be an expression of total gift – total gift of the whole person, where we yield up all that we are to the other, confident of the total receiving by the other. This total giving and receiving is the point where man and woman can experience the deepest sense of union, accepting and embracing, as it does, all dimensions of their manhood and womanhood, including the procreative dimension. Any withholding, whether mental, emotional or physical, diminishes the meaning of the act.

Any way we choose to manage fertility will, inevitably, affect the unitive/personal aspect of intercourse, either for better or for worse.

If we abstract the procreative element in intercourse and attempt to deal with it alone, we encourage an attitude to fertility that sees it as a problem rather than as the healthy, desirable and integral part of human sexuality that it is. Attitudes towards it become the same as attitudes towards any medical problem – get the expert to treat it, or remove it. By meeting it in the context of the total sexual expression, we encourage couples to grow in their understanding and experience of the unitive side of intercourse, as well as of the unitive side of their whole relationship, which will, automatically, improve their responses to their needs and hopes on the procreative front.

Natural family planning opens us to methods of fertility management which have the possibility of holding the whole man and woman, the whole act of giving and receiving and the whole pleasure and goodness of sexual communication under God.

Problems in Practice

Some problems in practice arise from the fact that intercourse is not always experienced as it is meant to be. Couples enter marriage with their own personal histories that have formed them and the limitations imposed on them by attitudes learned from childhood. Even today, one meets people whose attitude to their bodies and to sex is that these are unclean, unholy. Intercourse, for them, is anything but healthy, good and uniting, and they bear the burden of more babies that they would choose as the only way of rationalising this 'distasteful' act.

Many women learn from their mothers, who have apparently enjoyed little of the unitive side of sex, that intercourse is something husbands expect and have a right to. It is the price one pays for being married. They bring to intercourse a sense of duty that is, in fact, strong enough to motivate them to initiate it when pregnancy may result, even though the menfolk themselves may be willing to abstain.

On the other hand, the threat of pregnancy itself may be used to manipulate the sexual expression in a relationship. Many women use it as a means of avoiding intercourse. That they want to avoid intercourse is indicative that the affective/unitive experience is absent. Intercourse, for these women, may be experienced as a way of being used, not necessarily due to any ill-will or abuse on the husband's part, but through his personal limitations imposed by poor education in relationships and ignorance of the real meaning of good sex.

A genuine fear of pregnancy is also a problem that arises frequently. This fear can build up to pathological proportions. It is not unknown for us to receive calls from women seeking reassurance, even though total abstinence is being practised. Their reason tells them they cannot possibly be pregnant and yet, so great is their anxiety, reason cannot overcome it.

As far as we can gather, one of the most common factors in the cause of profound anxiety about pregnancy is a bad experience of childbirth. This 'bad experience' is related in terms of difficult labour accompanied by what the clients experience as insensitive handling by the personnel involved. Women feeling such anxiety are often mistrustful of any method of family planning. Their fear invades the unitive dimension of sexual expression, causing them to view intercourse itself as a threat, and can affect their whole response to their partner, ultimately seeing the person of their husband as threatening.

It is surprising the numbers of such clients who are critical of the attitudes of doctors and nurses in maternity hospitals. I realise that childbirth, indeed any stay in hospital, is grist for the gossip mill and, like the fisherman, women are prone to capping the previous story. However, one cannot completely dismiss experiences that have obviously deeply affected attitudes to further pregnancy and to the hospitals themselves.

Another situation which arises in practice is that of the couple who seek family planning advice and information but their whole life-style militates against implementing it. These couples have difficulty taking control of any aspect of their lives – again, probably, because of their personal histories and background. Planning is an alien concept for them and, while natural family planning may well be an introduction to taking responsibility on themselves, one must be conscious of the conversion required and the possible consequences in such cases. By conversion, I mean a whole change of attitude leading them to begin to plan when they will have intercourse and when they will not; to take on the discipline of keeping a chart; and to look hard at the decision about whether or not they want to avoid another baby.

Finally, on this point, there is the problem of motivation. What does each individual couple really mean when they say they want to avoid a pregnancy? Do they want to avoid one at any cost, at some cost, or is it likely they will turn round, in midstream, taking risks because another value has become more important? Are they being honest with you, their partner or themselves? Experience indicates this to be one of the really grey areas that causes one to acknowledge the complexities of human behaviour and response.

At a very straightforward level, one may find oneself facing a client anxious to know whether there is the possibility of pregnancy or not. When the moment of confirmation that she is not pregnant arrives, why, so often, the barely disguised crestfallenness? Why the rampant grin on a husband's face when pregnancy is confirmed, even though he has previously impressed you with the need to avoid such an event?! More seriously, it would seem to me, pregnancy can be a massive statement where other efforts at communication have failed; for example, in indicating a partner's dissatisfaction with the method of family planning being used or, indeed, dissatisfaction with intercourse, or the domestic environment.

Pregnancy, even when apparently not desired, can be a form of withdrawal. This is, as yet, a rather tentative suggestion. A woman expecting a baby is in a special state; a world a little apart, where she may feel somewhat released or excused from facing the grim realities of her life. The realities remain, and the new baby may well add to them, but are they muffled somewhat by her condition, and by the response that this draws forth from others?

These are only some of the problem areas encountered in practice which demonstrate that simple solutions to fertility control are not always adequate to meet the total needs of couples who seek help. Our own expertise is improved by the growing awareness and understanding of the various factors that can influence couples' responses to intercourse, fertility and pregnancy. Each couple who comes to us contributes to the help we can give to the couple who follows.

Natural Family Planning

As stated earlier, a good method of family planning is not simply one that is effective in preventing pregnancy. Total abstinence will certainly achieve that but we could hardly call it a good method! A good method must be effective in enabling a couple to plan their babies but it must also be one that promotes love, harmony, and is supportive of the unitive aspect of intercourse. It must be acceptable to the couple at the moral level. It must not be detrimental to the health of either partner. It must be aesthetically acceptable and must not cause anxiety.

Natural family planning methods can be as effective in avoiding pregnancy as any of the contraceptive methods, and more effective than some, provided they are well taught and well understood, and that the couple are willing to take responsibility for their fertility. For a couple to take on this responsibility themselves is a very important factor in growth and maturity. We are inclined to tremble at the thought of the couple taking their fertility into their own hands, especially if we perceive their need to avoid a pregnancy as considerable. Yet it seems a pity that often the real value of a couple's decision to manage their fertility from within, as opposed to a solution imposed from without by use of contraceptives, is so underestimated.

The use of natural family planning calls for mutual cooperation between partners, which is why, ideally, it is so important to try and meet the couple together rather than the wife alone. In meeting the couple together, first they are shown how fertility is shared. Surprisingly enough, this is a perception that is often absent, and the demonstration of this simple fact can be enough to motivate a reluctant husband.

Embarking on the use of these methods, couples are encouraged to communicate with one another about the presence or absence of signs of fertility in the wife. As the demands of abstinence are explored with them, couples are invited to communicate to one another their feelings about intercourse, their fears, their personal needs, their feelings about the possibility of pregnancy and what this might mean for them individually and as a family. This is communication at a most intimate and personal level and, frequently, we find it is the first genuine communication that has taken place for a long time in some marriages. This has a most positive effect on the relationship, the fruits of which may spread into other areas of their lives together.

Natural family planning methods are acceptable at the moral level. Couples may use methods that one or other of them find morally unacceptable and this creates tension between them. Even those couples who state they have sorted the moral problem out for themselves may not be as much at peace as they seem. Occasionally, one finds that the sorting out has privately involved a kind of quid pro quo deal. . . . 'We/I will use contraception because I feel it is necessary and/or because I have been told I ought to, or may, and, in return, I will refrain from receiving the Eucharist', almost as though not receiving the Eucharist were a sacrifice for the use of contraception. In some such cases, it may be that these couples or individual spouses should be helped to a real peace in continuing with their family planning arrangements but, in others, the only way of relieving anxiety is to show them a method that is approved morally and help them towards an implementation of it in a way that will meet their needs.

Natural family planning methods do not damage health. This is an important consideration, especially as people are more aware than ever before of the risks attached to the use of some of the other methods. I do not propose to explore the more obvious physical ill-effects. However, any method that causes anxiety about health is damaging to the relationship, as the cause of the anxiety quickly becomes transferred, for example, from the 'pill' to the person of the partner. So, the spouse who is concerned about the possible risks to health, or to fertility, or to the health of future children, by the use of particular methods, may view the whole question of sex, in all its dimensions, as burden rather than gift.

Natural family planning methods are aesthetically acceptable. They enable a couple to have intercourse in the way God and Nature intended – unadorned, except with their own love and desire. Although there are those who do not have any difficulties, aesthetically speaking, with other methods, or who find other values outweigh the aesthetic one, there are many for whom the experience of pleasure and goodness in sex can be greatly diminished by the method they use.

These are all values which are involved in good family planning. It is not enough that we are aware of them ourselves. We have a role to play in educating couples seeking guidance, in order that the choices they make will be informed and the decisions they take will be based not only on the quantity of intercourse they may have through use of a particular method but on the quality of intercourse some methods can bring.

Abstinence

Natural family planning involves in its use the practice of abstinence. Couples using these methods are limited to the infertile times of each cycle if they wish to avoid pregnancy. This calls for a discipline and control that other methods do not demand.

Abstinence, undoubtedly, is one of the real difficulties for many with the use of natural methods. However, I think we should try and get it into perspective. Many of the couples who seek natural family planning have already been practising abstinence to a heroic degree, and are more than happy with what natural family planning can offer them. Again, there are couples who have used withdrawal as a way of controlling fertility, conceiving all their children along the way, and who have never, or rarely, known complete and relaxed intercourse. For them, too, the discovery of the infertile period can seem like riches indeed. Nevertheless, for many, abstinence and its integration as part of positive sexual behaviour calls for conversion, and we must be realistic with couples about the demands it may make.

I think it can be helpful for couples if abstinence can be demonstrated as a normal part of married love, and I would like to quote here from an article of my own which touched on this point:

> Intercourse is an act of love – of love that is responsive to the needs of the individual, the couple and the family. However, apart from fertility control, there are many occasions within a marriage when it may not be appropriate to express this loving response, which leads one to ask is abstinence a normal and natural part of positive sexual expression? For example, there are times when refraining from intercourse may be desirable, or even necessary, during a pregnancy which is threatened. In this situation, abstinence is the caring response to the child in the womb and to the hopes of the couple for that child. Refraining from intercourse for a period after childbirth is usually desirable, and this is in no way seen as detrimental to a couple's loving response to each other. Illness, too, makes its own demands on couples to care for one another in a way that precludes intercourse. At less dramatic levels, there are many instances in a marriage where abstinence is involved; when partners are separated by work or family situations. This does not even begin to take account of all the times couples choose not to avail of intercourse simply because they do not wish to. And in no way are these abstinences seen or experienced as detracting from the value and importance of intercourse to the relationship; nor do couples experience themselves as less loving, less responsive or less sexually motivated because of it.
>
> It would appear from this that in these life situations, there is an ongoing judgment as to whether it is appropriate for a couple to express their feelings through intercourse or through abstaining from intercourse, and that this appropriateness is largely responsible for satisfaction in either event. No doubt, there are times in all of these situations when a couple will look at one another and deeply wish they need not refrain, but accept it as part of living and loving together, and the wish itself is an affirmation of one another and of intercourse.
>
> Arriving at a realisation that abstinence is a normal part of married love is one of the first steps towards successful use of natural family planning. However, one must be sensitive to what may be reasonably expected from couples in this regard. There is a balance within the norm. If abstinence is almost the total experience of sexual expression, then it may be an abnormal and unnatural situation for the couple. There may be no easy solution for the couple requesting natural family planning advice where the husband's work permits him to be at home only two nights in a fortnight, or where husband and wife are both doing shift work.[1]

At the same time, abstinence from intercourse does not mean abstinence from loving or from any form of sexual expression. One of the positive aspects of a method of family planning which requires that a couple refrain from intercourse periodically is that it can invite and, indeed, encourage a much broader experience of affective communication while, at the same time, enhancing the value and meaning for the couple of intercourse when it can be experienced. Abstinence can highlight that sexual tautness between man and woman; can heighten their awareness of one another and their desire for one another. In a world where many spouses express feelings of neglect or inattention, or feel themselves to be no more than an ignored cog in a big machine, this awareness can be very affirmative of their person. In this context, couples are encouraged to experience all the ways and the values of sexual loving outside of intercourse that they find appropriate to their particular relationship.

Abstinence itself is not necessarily a limitation in a method of family planning, but the amount required from couple to couple may well be. With increasing knowledge and research into identifying the actual limits of the fertile period, I would hope this time may be greatly reduced for most couples. This would certainly alter certain negative responses to natural family planning and ease the particular burden abstinence places on some couples. Nevertheless, the task will still remain of helping men and women to develop and grow towards a healthy, joyful and generous appreciation of the gift and meaning of their sexuality.

Limitations of Natural Family Planning: Contraception

There are those who would claim that natural family planning has no limitations. However, we know, in practice, that there are many for whom a natural method of family planning would be either inappropriate or unworkable. For example, there are many women who bear the burden of spouses who drink heavily or whose consideration for them is minimal. In addition, they are open, unfortunately, to abuse at the sexual level which may result in more pregnancies and children than they can cope with.

There are also women who find it extremely difficult to detect a clear pattern of fertility and infertility. This may be due to over-anxiety about becoming pregnant or about the method of family planning in use. It may be due to hidden factors which will surface only with difficulty. Or it may be due, simply, to the fact that some women cannot recognise such a pattern. There are couples like those mentioned earlier, whose whole training in life militates against their taking on the disciplines of natural family planning, and for some of whom, the avoidance of a pregnancy might be critical; those whose life situations impose a far greater degree of abstinence than might be consistent with good marriage and those who simply cannot bring themselves to trust these methods.

How can we help these people? Can contraception? (I exclude any kind of abortifacient contraception from these considerations.) From the point of view of good family planning, which should contain all the qualities and respect all the values mentioned at the beginning, contraception cannot be seen as good. However, I think it is important that we listen carefully to the experience of those who say that they have found contraception of some help at a particular time. Frequently, couples or individual spouses who have used contraception at particular points in their marriage speak of the way it has enabled them to weather a very difficult phase. With hindsight, and even at the time indeed, they are aware of the limitations of such an approach to their fertility and sexual expression, but they are also conscious of the needs of a particular time and the values they were trying to preserve, for which contraception appeared to be, at least in their eyes, the only answer in a difficult situation. For these reasons, it would seem to me that contraception may have a limited role to play in helping these people with their marriages and family relationships in an overall sense and can provide what may be the vital space necessary for them to grow towards the ideal, provided that the helping agency is firmly committed to that aim. (It is interesting to note that couples seldom enthuse about contraceptives but rather acknowledge them as perhaps the only answer in a particular situation.) When we meet such persons and enter into the realities of their position which seems to preclude, for the moment anyway, the use of natural family planning, part of our encouragement in growth towards the ideal can be positive acceptance of the reality which they experience and an attitude on our part which is supportive in decisions which they believe to be right for them.

Natural family planning demands certain qualities in a relationship before it can be feasible. By turning our backs when these qualities are absent, or have not yet developed, often through no fault of the persons concerned, we forfeit the opportunity to positively help them. They will either return to their families confirmed in their anxieties or they will seek help from agencies whose convictions differ from our own.

Goodness and wholeness are the goals we all aspire to. We are each at a different stage on the journey towards them. If we look at natural family planning as contributing to these goals, it may be possible to see the provision of contraception, in certain cases, as useful in coping with a particular inadequacy for a time, with a view to building up and on the strengths and potential present. By so doing, and by continuing to hold the persons concerned in our care, we respond responsibly to their present reality and to our hopes for their future.

I am conscious that in these remarks is reflected my own application of an ideal which sees natural family planning as desirable, and which intends natural family planning to be the goal of any counselling strategy. Concepts such as 'personal growth', 'gradualness' and 'progress towards the ideal' would not, I think, exclude the kind of acceptance of situations which is suggested here. These concepts and this type of strategy, I feel, serve the interests not only of good morals but of good medicine.

Family Planning Counselling

In my view, the ideal family planning facility is one which has as its prime concern the teaching of natural family planning in a way that educates couples in the autonomous control of their fertility as a positive approach to good sex and good relationship. The commitment to natural family planning must be wholehearted, and this is where we must emphasise the importance of our own confidence in the effectiveness of these methods. Doctors and nurses, in the attitudes they show to their patients, can have an enormous influence in either encouraging or discouraging couples in this respect. They are authority figures and ones in whom the public place a lot of confidence.

Such a facility should be able to provide accurate information on all methods of family planning, including contraceptive methods. Frequently, couples make bad choices simply because they are not fully informed. This information should include not only the advantages and limitations of the methods but also the modification in sexual behaviour they require, be it for the use of natural methods or the use of contraceptives.

The approach should be a counselling approach. Good instruction on charting etc. is essential, but as I have here tried to show, if a couple are to be really helped and the management of fertility is to contribute to the health and well-being of the whole relationship, it is necessary to enter into that relationship, with the couple, exploring with them where the strengths and weakness for them may lie in relation to the method they are choosing. Actually, by alerting a couple at this stage to these issues, a lot of difficulties can be avoided.

In this respect, a critical factor in a good family planning service is the kind of person recruited to provide it and the type of training they are given.

With regard to doctors themselves providing a service in family planning, I can see practical difficulties, if only at the time level. Ideally, I think, in a hospital situation, there should be a service staffed by competent teachers which would be a resource used by the doctors – not as a place to hive off patients, but as part of the continuing care of doctor for patient, with a three-way dynamic between doctor, patient and teacher.

Doctors in group practice could certainly consider employing the services of a family planning teacher in their surgeries, even on a one day a week basis. This may be possible also for a doctor in single practice or he could, perhaps, link up with such services provided locally, if they exist.

A family planning facility should also see itself as a possible referral agency. Because of the nature of fertility problems and the kind of relationship that exists between teacher and client, problems other than those directly linked with fertility frequently emerge. For example, it may become evident that there is a psycho-sexual problem involved, or a gynaecological one, an alcoholic one or problems in the relationship itself. Where it seems that a client would welcome help in these areas too, we should, with the client's permission, call on other resources available, bearing in mind that our service is to the health and happiness of the whole person or couple.

The other side of the coin is shown when fertility guidance helps couples to achieve pregnancy. This may come about through simply educating couples in identifying their most fertile time. However, where there is a problem of infertility, we should be able to direct couples to the best help available.

I have dealt here with some aspects of the personal factors involved in family planning. There has been no mention, for example, of the whole area where good counselling might be the encouragement needed by some couples to have a baby; or of those attitudes to fertility and to children which respond to the kind of society in which we live.

It is worth indicating, finally, the broad perspective needed for an overall view. Family planning swings right across the spectrum – from those who seem to have everything under control, including the 'statutory' two children, to those who seem to have nothing under control. In considering what good family planning is, we must consider what good family is and, specifically, what good planning and good family are for each individual family community.

8

Medico-moral Problems in the Management of Congenital Malformation

EDWARD GUINEY

Approximately two per cent of all babies are born with a significant life-threatening congenital malformation. Some of these are not amenable to treatment and the infant dies soon after birth. Of those which are treatable, the treatment, usually surgical, frequently completely corrects the abnormality and the infant has a normal life expectancy with full potential for intellectual and physical development. This happy outcome would be often seen following surgical correction of neonatal intestinal obstruction.

Unfortunately in other infants, although the immediate threat to life may be removed by medical or surgical intervention, the infant is permanently disabled by the consequences of the defects which have been established in utero. With treatment such infants may survive, but do so as inevitably handicapped, sometimes both intellectually and physically. This situation is most frequently met in babies born with spina bifida.

The management of such inevitably permanently disabled infants is the focal point of much present-day controversy. Many experts, particularly amongst doctors responsible for the care of these infants, question the rectitude of treating all such babies in a comprehensive manner. It is recommended and so practised in many centres, that those infants with serious permanent malformations should not be treated actively, and that no effort should be made to prolong their lives. The application of this principle is well illustrated in the present-day management of spina bifida. This congenital abnormality has been central in concentrating the thoughts of doctors and moralists on the whole issue of ethical implications in the care of the congenitally malformed.

Spina bifida is an abnormality as a result of which the infant is born with a defect in the spinal column. As a consequence of the defect the function of the spinal cord is impaired. Many such infants are born with total absence of sensation and paralysis of their lower limbs and with a lack of control of their bladder and back passage. This means that as they grow they will never be able to walk without artificial support, will in many cases be confined to a wheelchair and will have double incontinence.

In addition the abnormality is usually accompanied by hydrocephalus, which itself is frequently associated with intellectual impairment.

It is possible at birth to identify infants who, if they live, will undoubtedly have lower limb paralysis and double incontinence. It is also possible to state that the great majority (75 per cent approximately) of those infants so identified will have an intelligence quotient of less than 80 and will frequently be severely mentally retarded.

Prior to 1970 there was great enthusiasm in many centres for treating all infants with spina bifida with equal intensity. As a result of this approach there emerged a small surviving population of extremely physically and intellectually handicapped children, which provoked an analysis and re-assessment of this unquestioning policy of intensive care.

Powerful modern techniques and drugs are available to doctors today to sustain and prolong life. Does the fact that such powerful therapy is now available mean that it must necessarily be offered to every patient, irrespective of the long-term prognosis for physical and intellectual development of each individual?

Because of the experience gained in the management of spina bifida prior to 1970, many paediatricians now believe strongly that availability of a treatment does not bring an obligation to apply or use it in all cases of congenital malformation. This principle is generally accepted in medicine when considering terminal painful illness of the elderly, or those who through an accident have acquired irreparable brain damage. Should it not also apply in the case of the newborn?

A policy of selection is now widely proposed and in fact, practised in some centres in the management of spina bifida. This implies that following birth, those infants identified as having very severe malformations will not be actively treated. This decision is made in the realisation that the withholding of the treatment is likely to result in the early death of the infant, an eventuality which those who accept and apply the policy of selection believe to be preferable to prolongation of the life of a severely handicapped individual.

Doctors universally accept that it is their duty to preserve life and alleviate suffering. When the preservation of life inevitably results in the prolongation of suffering, then the doctor must question which of these duties takes precedence. The answer to this problem will vary with circumstances, and will certainly be influenced by how strenuous the efforts needed to prolong life are, and how great the suffering may be which the patient has to endure in his extended life.

Those doctors who support a policy of selection in the care of spina bifida do so in the belief that it is not a part of their function to actively prolong the life of an infant who will inevitably have absence of sensation and total motor paralysis of its lower limbs as well as incontinence of urine and faeces and, often, intellectual impairment.

This is not an intellectual abstraction on the part of the doctor. The suffering of such infants was seen, and continues to be seen in the survivors of the regime of treatment of the 1960s which did not countenance selection. It is the misery of many of these infants which has impelled so many paediatricians and paediatric surgeons to support and apply a selective policy. Many would feel that not to select represents professional irresponsibility. In seeking to explain, and when challenged to justify, selection, doctors find that they have to vocalise and define why their estimate of a patient's potential suffering leads them to withhold life-prolonging measures. It is at this point that the doctor begins to use phrases such as 'quality of life', which lead on to value judgments of another person's life, and explanations that an individual's inevitable handicaps are 'incompatible with human dignity, contentment and happiness'.

These phrases and these concepts are beyond the usual field of competence of doctors, who feel uneasy and fearful when discussing them. The medical profession has sought guidance on the ethical acceptability of these phrases and concepts, from experts, especially religious commentators and moral theologians.

When a decision regarding the management of an infant is made, the doctor plays an active and indeed dominant role. Why should this be so? Is the doctor's dominant role inevitable or desirable?

With regard to the disabled infant there are three possible participants in the decision-making process: the parents, the doctors, and society through its courts and legislature.

It would seem obvious that the parents of the infant have the greatest moral authority and interest in making a decision for or against treatment. The ideal is that the parents, having been expertly and dispassionately informed of the medical condition and prognosis by the doctors, should then decide how they wish the malformed infant be treated. Unfortunately, the ideal of well-informed, objective involvement of the parents is not easily attained.

The parents cannot be dispassionate, or objective. They are emotionally deeply involved and psychologically under great strain as a result of the birth of their malformed infant. If they have the intellectual training and ability to understand the issues explained to them, they frequently recoil from making life or death decisions regarding their child. It is unfair and irresponsible in these circumstances for the doctors to force parents to decide. Any decision they make may be one they subsequently regret. Most frequently the parents will say they wish the doctor to advise them positively, and to do that which he feels best for the babe. The doctor is the expert, and that is why he is in attendance. He must accept the responsibilities of the expert. The doctor's expertise is by skilful compassionate explanation to lead the parents to acquiesce in what he believes to be the correct course of action. The author does not agree, as some suggest, that it is possible to present parents with an audit of the situation and then leave them to make up their own minds.

A further problem in relation to the parents as decision-makers, is the fact that quite frequently they are not available to discuss the problem. This is particularly true in the case of the mother, who may be confined in a maternity hospital many miles from the central unit to which the neonate has been urgently transferred. This geographic difficulty may also apply to the father. The optimum time to treat many of these infants, particularly in the case of spina bifida, is as soon as possible after birth, and consequently the combination of pressure of time and distance of parents from the hospital may mean that the ideal lengthy and, if necessary, repeated conversations between the doctor and the parents are not feasible.

If the doctor is to play a dominant role in decision-making, it is essential that he does so in consultation with his colleagues, that a medical team be involved and that the team be expert and knowledgeable about the prognosis and treatment of the malformation.

Let us consider the role of the courts and lawyers in decision-making. If rules of behaviour or a legally enforceable code of practice are laid down, it is inevitable that the freedom of parents and doctors to take responsible and informed decisions will be severely curtailed. At first sight this curtailment may seem to be what society wants; protection against 'the doctor playing God', but it would eliminate rational judgment and medical experience from the decision-making process. Legislation or rules of conduct which were enforced by legal penalties would mean suspension of medical and even parental judgment, and treatment might often be instituted, dictated by self-protection or fear of punishment, rather than by the primary interest of the patient.

As it is indicated in the preceding paragraphs, the circumstances surrounding the birth of a malformed infant are such that the medical people are frequently forced into making fundamental decisions regarding the prolongation or otherwise of the life of the infant. The doctor's primary expertise is in sickness and health and not in the making of such decisions. He may not want the responsibility of making decisions regarding the giving or withholding of life-supporting care. However, in the absence of any other decision-maker the doctor is forced to assume that role. If he is to continue to do so to the benefit of his patients, it will be in the context of a vigilant concerned society rather than in a legally constrained potentially punitive environment.

There is controversy among moralists and other commentators and experts regarding the ethical acceptance of a selective policy of treatment for the congenitally malformed. Those responsible for the care of such infants – that is, the doctors and nursing personnel, must work out a policy of management in the context of the outlook and views of the society in which they work. This evolved policy must be ethically and legally acceptable to the authorities and people of the country in which it is being applied.

In some states of the United States a selective policy is not legally permissible, while in Great Britain such a policy seems to be readily accepted, as is the hastening of the death of the non-treated infants by sedation and sub-caloric feeding.

It appears that between these two extremes another way may be identified which requires neither that all infants be treated nor countenances a form of euthanasia.

It is not difficult to argue in favour of a selective policy when one considers the medical facts. However, it is difficult to produce an irrefutable justification from the viewpoint of ethics. This is not to suggest that the medical and ethical positions are disparate, they are but limbs of the same body.

To discuss ethics we must use the terminology of ethics. This implies that we consider the terms, ordinary and extraordinary means. It is generally accepted that while one must always use ordinary means to support life one need not always apply extraordinary means. When we seek to define ordinary and extraordinary means, we find that the definitions are not clear cut and distinct. They are subject to interpretation. Nevertheless, if we accept that ordinary means are those which:

(i) promise recovery, either from present condition of illness, or from general grave condition associated with handicap,

(ii) do not place a great burden on the patient with no realistic hope of good prognosis,

then it can be held that full-scale active intervention for the severely malformed and inevitably handicapped is extraordinary means, and consequently means which those in attendance are not bound to use.

If we do accept selection, there are certain difficult consequences deriving from selection itself which need to be examined. We select with the intention of minimising suffering and we do so in the expectation and anticipation of the early death of the infant. It is therefore contrary to the very purpose of selection to treat the death-causing complications which appear in the infants. For example, infection, particularly meningitis, is a very common cause of death in untreated spina bifida infants. If we accept selection we should not treat the infection since to do so is in direct conflict with the whole basis of selection and its intention. Even harder to accept, but still as logical, is that if such infants commence vomiting, they should not be given intravenous fluids or feeding, since to do so is once again to prolong life. In these circumstances, intravenous fluids constitute extraordinary means.

If selection is accepted, then the policy must be that no active therapeutic step will be taken which might prolong the life of the child, and, of equal importance, no intentional measure directly or indirectly aimed at shortening the infant's life may be permitted. The infant shall however have full custodial care, warmth, change of clothing and full caloric feeding.

There are many objections to the policy of selection. Three of the most powerful are:

(i) that an error in selection may be made;

(ii) that a selected infant may not die;

(iii) that the decision is a proxy one made on behalf of a non-consenting individual, the new-born infant.

The first of these objections suggests that an erroneous selection could mean that a potentially perfect or minimally handicapped infant was rejected for treatment. In particular with regard to the intelligence of the infant it is impossible to refute this objection. It is because of the possibility of error and in an effort to obviate it that the selection must be made by an expert or team of experts, in full knowledge of the medical status of the infant and of the known prognosis of the malformation.

The objection that a selected infant may not die implies that not only may the child survive indefinitely, but that it will be more handicapped than it would have been if it had been treated initially. Indeed it is this argument which has led some who accept selection to accept mercy killing of those infants who are not treated. These two objections are powerful, and while they can be strongly countered they cannot be totally refuted. I do not believe that because of the arguments against it the whole selective policy is untenable. There is a possibility of error in every activity and most certainly in day-to-day medical care. As experts, doctors in full knowledge make judgments and choices. The fact that the choice is not always correct, does not imply that because of fear of error judgment and choice should be suspended.

In this regard however, it is important that not only should the decision or selection be an expert one, to minimise error, but also that those in charge should keep an open mind regarding reversal of the choice. This may occur because the baby thrives, because the parents wish for active management, or because it becomes obvious that an infant will live indefinitely while experiencing suffering which can be alleviated by intervention.

With reference to the problem that the decision not to treat is a proxy one, imposed on a non-consenting individual by a person or persons who judge the value of another's life by their own criteria, there is again no satisfactory rebuttal of this argument. If one believes in selection, one believes that such a proxy decision is permissible and indeed desirable.

Finally while the discussion in this article has focused on spina bifida, the medical/ethical problems arise in relation to many other congenital abnormalities such as Down's syndrome, congenital heart disease, cystic fibrosis etc. These are titles or descriptive terms, which embrace individuals, and it is on the basis of each individual and his/her quantum and potential for health, that selection may be hesitatingly applied. Selection if accepted and applied must be individualised, it must always relate to a particular patient. It must be seen for what it is, the most important decision in the life of an individual, and the decision-makers, whoever they may be, must always be aware of the awful responsibility of their role.

I have confined the discussion in this article to medico-moral problems consequent on a policy of selection based on the predicted physical and intellectual handicap of a newborn. As doctors we feel we can predict in this way, and reluctantly accept that selection is a necessary responsible consequence from such prognostication.

I have not sought or indeed dared to discuss here the non medical factors in a newborn's circumstances which may influence his ability to achieve his full potential for physical and intellectual development, limited though that may be as a consequence of the congenital abnormality. Clearly a disabled newborn who has been abandoned by its parents has much less chance of achieving human contentment and happiness than a similar infant taken into a loving parental home. What influence, if any, should such non-medical social factors have on selection? For the doctors: no influence; since, were it otherwise, we would really be moving outside our field of competence. Nevertheless, if value judgments are accepted as a basis for selection based on health factors, then the influence of social factors on these value judgments cannot be ignored by the moralists and society. The social factors will never go away even in the most opulent society. The moralists must consider how social factors extraneous to the patient may relate to the ordinariness or extraordinariness of a particular form of treatment. So, for example, the same treatment may be ordinary for patient A since his parents want him, and extraordinary for patient B since he has been rejected. Parents of A may be wealthy and capable of giving A great physical and affective support which will make his handicap supportable and compatible with contentment, while in case B physical and affective impoverishment seem assured with the inevitable accompanying misery.

It is not acceptable to the decision-makers to be told that these factors are irrelevant and even dangerous to consider. It is indeed true that once considered and vocalised as relevant, we are again on a new 'slippery slope' but unless efforts are made we shall never reach the top of the slope, and when we do there will be others there before us who have found non-acceptable ways of arriving there.

ADDITIONAL READING

Bioethics, New York: Paulist Press 1976.

Campbell, A.G.M. and Duff, R.S., 'Deciding the care of severely malformed or dying infants', *Journal of Medical Ethics*, 5 (1979), 65–7.

Duff, R.S. and Campbell, A.G.M., 'Moral and ethical dilemmas in the special care nursery', *The New England Journal of Medicine*, 289 (1973), 890–94.

Guiney, E.J., 'A question of Priorities', *Journal of the Irish Medical Assoc.*, 66 (1973), 401.
Lorber, J., *Devel. Med. Child. Neurol.*, 13 (1971), 279.
Swinyard, C.H., ed., *Decision Making and the Defective Newborn: Proceedings of a Conference on Spina Bifida and Ethics*, Springfield, Ill.: C.C. Thomas.

9

Ethical Issues in Reproductive Medicine: A Legal Perspective

WILLIAM BINCHY

The subject of this discussion is of very broad dimensions, and I can hope to deal with only some of its most important aspects.

Four principal areas will be covered: these are contraception, abortion, sterilisation and artificial insemination. Although these areas differ widely from one another in some respects, it is, I think, fair to say that they share some important common legal themes. I intend, later, to refer briefly to this common legal philosophy.

As will soon be clear, many of even the most basic of legal questions have never come before the Irish courts, so one can only speculate on how they would be determined. The problem is compounded by the fact that some of these questions really raise issues of moral and social policy, albeit clothed in judicial language. The task of analysis, therefore, is as much a matter of predicting the likely effect of the personal values of the judges on their judgment as it is of applying legal rules to a legal problem.

Contraception

Turning, therefore, to the first of these topics, contraception. This is a subject which has been endlessly debated and analysed in this country over the past decade, so I do not intend to retrace its history in great detail. I will instead look more towards the future than the past.

In order to discuss the future, it is, however, necessary to refer very briefly to previous events. As you know, until 1973, there was a total statutory prohibition on the sale or importation into Ireland of contraceptives. However, in the famous decision of *McGee* v *Attorney General,* [1] the Supreme Court held that the provision prohibiting the importation of contraceptives other than for sale was contrary to the Constitution.

The Constitution, of course, said nothing about contraception. Nor did it say anything about the right of marital privacy. What it did refer to was merely 'the personal rights of the citizen'. For three of the judges in *McGee,* this general reference to unspecified personal rights was sufficient to protect a right to marital privacy. These judges provided no clear analysis of the precise meaning and scope of this concept. Clearly it extended to the decision of a married couple to practise contraception. Beyond that it is impossible to know what the concept involves.

The Supreme Court in *McGee* was probably affected by the constitutional developments in the United States where, only eight years previously,[2] the United States Supreme Court had discovered the right of marital privacy which it defined in similarly vague terms. We will be looking in more detail shortly at how the concept of marital privacy was transformed in the United States into something very different from what it first appeared to be.

Whilst three of the judges in *McGee* regarded the right to marital privacy as one of the personal rights of the citizen, Judge Walsh, the other judge in the majority, considered that marital privacy was an aspect of the family rights conferred by a different Article in the Constitution. This difference of opinion is important for the future, since it may well affect the determination of a question which we will be considering in a few moments, namely whether unmarried persons have a constitutional right of access to contraceptives.

After *McGee*, as is well known, various attempts were made to resolve the unsatisfactory position resulting from the partial striking down of the original legislation. There seems no need to go through the history of the unsuccessful attempts at legislation. Let us therefore look briefly at the legislation which succeeded in making its way on to the statute-books – the Health (Family Planning) Act 1979.

The Act creates a right of access to contraceptives primarily in the context of family planning. A registered medical practitioner may give a prescription or authorisation for a contraceptive to a person if he is satisfied that the person 'is seeking the contraceptive, *bona fide*, for family planning purposes or for adequate medical reasons and in appropriate circumstances'.

Clearly, the object of the legislation is to provide for controlled access to contraceptives, so that they are not available as a matter of course to the unmarried and particularly to the younger members of our society. Equally clearly it would be impossible to accomplish this objective with complete success, and the legislation attempts to steer a middle course between strict rules as to entitlement and a general free-for-all. To what extent the Act will succeed in its purpose is a matter of controversy but there is little doubt that in its aim it would seem to have the support of the majority in our community.

The Act has, however, come under attack from a number of quarters, and there has been much talk of litigation attempting to have the Act struck down on constitutional grounds.

A wide range of possible grounds has already been mentioned. Let us consider one or two of them.

Denial of Access to Contraceptives for Married Persons

The first possible constitutional attack on the legislation might be that it is so drafted as to result in the denial of reasonable access to contraceptives for married persons.

It might be argued that it interferes with their constitutional right of privacy to require them to consult a doctor on a matter that is not essentially a medical one, and that to make their access to contraceptives depend on what subjective view the doctor may form on the question of their *bona fides* is unduly restrictive. Moreover, the effect of section 11 of the Act, which relieves any person from the obligation of giving prescriptions or selling contraceptives, may be that access to contraceptives will be somewhat limited, especially in some rural areas.

As against this, it can be argued that the legislation strikes a reasonable balance between a free-for-all in access to contraceptives, on the one hand, and undue restrictions, on the other. The fact that some couples may have greater difficulty than others in obtaining contraceptives is not in itself a reason for holding the Act unconstitutional.

In my view, whilst the resolution of this issue is by no means certain, the legislation is not likely to be struck down by our courts on this ground. (Whether the European Court of Human Rights would take another view is a separate question, which really goes beyond the scope of my remarks. I will say no more on it than that it is quite possible that the European Court would take a different view.)

Discrimination Against Unmarried Persons

The next constitutional argument against the legislation might be that it discriminates against unmarried persons by denying them access to contraceptives. A similar argument succeeded in the United States in 1972, where the Supreme Court held[3] that, since marital privacy affected two individuals – the husband and wife – really it involved an individual right which should attach also to single persons. This is, of course, highly questionable logic, and the decision cannot be defended on this ground.

Would it be followed here? I doubt it. The legislature is entitled to distinguish between people who are differently situated, and single people in this regard may be considered as different from married people. I have no doubt that the legislation has gone as far as it can to mitigate any harsh effects in respect of unmarried persons by permitting access to contraceptives to persons for *bona fide* purposes of family planning. In my view, the legislation would not be struck down on the basis of discrimination against the unmarried. The Court is permitted to have regard to the social and moral dimensions of the question. As Judge Griffin stated in *McGee:* 'in any ordered society the protection of morals through the deterrence of fornication and promiscuity is a legitimate legislative aim and a matter not of private but of public morality.'

The question is not, however, a closed one. If the Court were to regard the question as raising an issue of *private* rather than public morality, it would be faced with the difficult and somewhat unpredictable task of trying to determine whether access to contraceptives for unmarried persons would, in Judge Walsh's words in *McGee* 'injur[e] the common good'.

There are, of course, many other possible lines of attack on the constitutionality of the legislation: for example, that it discriminates against the poor in favour of those who can afford to go from Ireland to England and bring home contraceptives with them in their personal luggage; that the legislation interferes with the right to bodily integrity, or that it offends against the freedom of religion and conscience. Whether any of these attacks will succeed is difficult to predict but my general view of the legislation is that it is probably sufficiently malleable to withstand attack on the grounds of unconstitutionality.

The more likely attack on the legislation will almost certainly come from within the Oireachtas itself [the State Legislature. *Editor*], where we may predict that further pressure will be brought within a short period to extend the scope of access to contraception.

Abortion

Abortion has recently become a subject of public debate in this country. The best way of analysing its legal aspects appears to be to examine the questions of central importance raised by abortion – and some very important questions are raised – and then referring specifically to the context of the Irish law.

Is the Unborn Child a Person? The first question that the law might be expected to ask is whether an unborn child is a person. If he is, then it follows that he may not be killed without justification. Strangely this 'pivotal'[4] question has rarely been faced by the courts or legislatures. In England, for example, legislation in 1967 greatly extended the right to abortion with absolutely no reference in the statute to the issue of the child's status as a human being.[5] In the United States, the Supreme Court was faced with the issue in 1973.[6] It did not decide the question, however, holding instead that the unborn child was not a 'person' within the meaning of the Fourteenth Amendment of the United States Constitution (which contains the famous Equal Protection and Due Process Clauses). The fundamental philosophical question was thus avoided, the Court contending that, in view of the 'wide divergence of thinking on this most sensitive and difficult question', the state of Texas had acted unconstitutionally in 'adopting one theory of life [so as to] override the rights of the pregnant woman that are at stake'. Thus the Court, entirely on its own admission, failed to resolve what it called 'the difficult question of when life begins'.

This failure of either English or American law to resolve the basic question of the humanity of the unborn child must be criticised, whatever the true motives of the courts or legislature may be. If, on the one hand, there is a *genuine* reluctance to determine the issue, this may be criticised on the basis that the question is so fundamental that it requires to be resolved before any other subsidiary issues are determined. Moreover, a Court which is too timid to resolve such a basic moral issue could scarcely feel itself competent to determine other equally important moral questions in the legal forum.

If, on the other hand, the apparent failure to determine the issue amounts in reality to a decision that the unborn child is *not* a human being, then the courts and legislature should have the courage to say so clearly and be judged accordingly. From the standpoint of the child, the failure to resolve the issue of his humanity amounts in result to a finding that he is not a human being.

In striking contrast to the approach in England and the United States is that of the Constitutional Court of the Federal Republic of Germany in 1975.[7] The Court had no hesitation in holding that the German Constitution afforded protection to the unborn child's right of life.

The Constitution provided[8] that: 'Everyone has the right to life. . . . .'[9] The Court held that the protection afforded by this provision could:

> . . . not be limited either to the 'completed' human being after birth nor to the child about to be born which is independently capable of living. The right to life is guaranteed to everyone who 'lives'; no distinction can be made here between the various stages of life developing itself before birth, or between unborn and born life. Everyone in the sense of [the Constitutional provision] is 'everyone living'; expressed in another way: every life possessing human individuality; 'everyone' also includes the yet unborn human being.[10]

Why is there such a pronounced difference between the German approach and that favoured in England and the United States? The reason is historical. Germany can remember its recent past in which basic human values (including those in relation to the treatment of unborn children) were discarded.[11]

The Unborn Child's Legal Rights.[12] Until the rush to abortion in the past decade or so, the unborn child was the subject of an extensive and growing range of legal rights. He was given the same rights to inherit property as if he were already born. After initial hesitation,[13] the courts recognised his right to sue for injuries sustained before birth, at all events where he was subsequently born alive. Some courts in the United States went so far as to award damages even where the unborn child died before birth.

With the sudden legislation of abortion on demand, the legal rights of the unborn child had to be curtailed. Since the right to abortion was protected by constitutional or legislative decree, it took precedence over the legal rights of the unborn child. It is interesting, if futile, to speculate on what the position might have been had the development and extension of these legal rights continued for another decade before the right to abortion was asserted. It is possible that a different order of priorities might then have prevailed.

The Legislation of Abortion Based on Danger to the Mother's Health. The history of abortion law in most countries indicates a steady progression from prohibition through permission to abort based on the risk to the mother's life, to abortion based on the mother's health until finally abortion is regarded as a matter for the private decision of the mother, untrammelled by any social or medical consideration and unhindered by deference to any other person, including the father of the child.

The English experience is instructive. Until recently, abortion was prohibited by legislation which made it an offence punishable by life imprisonment for a pregnant woman or any other person to attempt to bring about the abortion of her child.[14]

In 1938, in the famous decision of *R.* v *Bourne*,[15] a doctor who had performed an abortion on a fourteen-year-old rape victim was prosecuted under this legislation. The doctor was at the time an advocate of more extensive abortion (although he has since become an eloquent opponent of abortion).

In instructing the jury, Mr Justice Macnaghten told them that it would be a defence to the charge if it could be shown that the abortion had been carried out to save the life of the mother. In this context, he stated:

> Life depends upon health, and it may be that health is so gravely impaired that death results . . . And if the probable consequence of the continuance of the pregnancy will be to make the woman a physical or mental wreck, the jury are quite entitled to take the view that the doctor who, in those circumstances, and in that honest belief, operates, is operating for the purpose of preserving the life of the woman.

Dr Bourne was acquitted, and his acquittal opened the door to still further extension of the law. The decision has been recognised by many commentators[16] (including those sympathetic to abortion)[17] as legally unsound. The concept of 'health' is obviously capable of extending far beyond life-and-death cases, on which it is ostensibly based.

The English Abortion Act of 1967 echoed in part the approach favoured in *Bourne*'s case by legalising an abortion on broad 'medical' grounds: an abortion will be legal where the risk of injury to the life or physical or mental health of a pregnant woman is greater than if the pregnancy were terminated; it may also be performed where there is a similar risk to the physical and mental health of any *existing children* of the woman's family.[18] In determining whether this risk exists, the doctors are permitted to take account of the mother's 'actual or reasonably foreseeable environment'.[19] Not surprisingly, these amorphous parameters of the notion of the woman's health have resulted in what is in fact (if not in strict legal theory) abortion on demand.[20]

Abortion Based on a Woman's Private Decision. The extension of the notion of risk to a woman's health contributed to the growth of the view that the woman herself should have a right to choose whether to remain pregnant. Since the medical role in this decision is merely to rubber stamp the woman's previous decision on the question, it has been argued that the reality rather than the form should be recognised by the law. But more important in this change of direction has been the growth of the new feminism, which stresses the autonomy of women in respect of reproduction. Strikingly absent from much feminist analysis is any marked concern for the determination of the issue of the humanity of the unborn child.

The Law has reflected this changing philosophy. Most notable are the developments in the United States.

In 1973, in *Roe* v *Wade*,[21] the United States Supreme Court held that the right of privacy was 'broad enough to encompass a woman's decision whether or not to terminate her pregnancy'. The Court did not regard the right of privacy as absolute: at some point after the first trimester the interests of the State concerning the protection of health, medical standards and prenatal life became dominant.

A number of problems result from the adoption of an analysis justifying abortion on the basis of a right to *privacy*. First, as has been mentioned, it forecloses consideration of the most important issue of the child's humanity. Secondly, it removes from scrutiny the moral and social dimensions in which the decision to abort is made. Thirdly, in stressing individual autonomy, it drives a wedge between mother and other persons (notably the father of the child) who might reasonably be regarded as having an interest in the child's welfare. Finally, if the right to privacy can justify abortion, it may also be involved in respect of other life-and-death decisions such as infanticide, euthanasia and suicide. What is originally regarded as a narrow issue of criminal law, therefore, involves far more wide-ranging social and legal implications.

Abortion Based on Child's 'Defectiveness'. Parallel with the growth of the concept of privacy as a justification of abortion has been the development of the notion that it is legally justifiable to abort a child who is likely to suffer from physical or mental 'defects'.[22] Still more ominously, abortion has been justified in respect of a child who, although perfectly healthy himself, may, when an adult, produce unhealthy children. Moreover, abortions have been carried out even in cases where the risk of injury is relatively slight.

The legal justification for this practice is difficult to discern. The practice compromises:

> what is surely one of the moral-legal absolutes of Anglo-American law – the principle that the life of an innocent human being may not be taken away simply because, in the judgment of society, non-life for this particular individual would be better than life.[23]

The legal implications of recognising defectiveness as a ground for abortion are alarming. First, if the *risk* of defectiveness is the basis of disentitlement to life, it can be argued that it is more sensible and, according to a somewhat perverse logic, more just, that abortion should be delayed until very late so as to be sure that the suspicions are correct and that healthy children are not unwittingly sacrificed. This argument was recently made in respectable medical circles in Britain during the debates on the Corrie Bill. The step to infanticide thus becomes a very small one in this context. It has been argued that the law should adopt a 'delayed personhood policy' in respect of 'defective' infants:

> This theory dictates that the state delay recognition of the child's personhood until the infant's potentiality for development has been established.[24] Adherents to this view argue that it would be namely an extension of the holding in *Roe* v *Wade*[25], which employed the fiction of non-personhood to obscure the reality of a rule change.[26]

The second implication in recognising defectiveness as a ground for abortion is that the perspective will shift (in fact if not in theory) from that of the *child's* interests to the interests of *others*. The 'tremendous cost to society of caring for retarded and congenitally malformed children'[27] has been identified as a factor to which legislators will have regard in determining whether abortion on this ground should be legally permissible. If social costs are to be the criterion of entitlement to life, it would be justifiable (and, indeed, arguably necessary) to abort children of the most deprived social groups, such as gypsies and racial minorities.[28]

Turning, then, to the Position in Ireland

The position in Ireland is that abortion is a criminal offence, under legislation enacted for Britain and Ireland in 1861.

There has been no litigation in this country in which the scope of this legislation has been analysed. It is therefore impossible to predict whether the English decision of *R.* v *Bourne*[29] (which we have already discussed) would be followed here. It will be recalled that that decision held that necessity was a defence to a prosecution for abortion, and that an abortion performed to save the life of the mother would thus be permissible. It seems that this part of the judgment would represent the law in this country. But where that judgment went on to hold that an abortion would be lawful if designed to save the mother from becoming a 'physical or mental wreck', this would surely not represent our law, since it goes far beyond what the defence of necessity can encompass.

The legislation of abortion in other countries has resulted in a number of women going from Ireland to these countries – mainly England – to have an abortion. It would seem that they do not commit an offence in doing so, since the crime of abortion is not extraterritorial. In other words, a prosecution for abortion must relate to an abortion committed in this country. Whether a woman could be convicted of *attempting* to have an abortion – which is a crime here – by setting in motion a plan to have an abortion in England is doubtful in the extreme. The law relating to attempts tends to require proof of a virtually completed act rather than mere preparation, even if that preparation clearly points to the intended commission of the offence.

Similarly it does not seem that a person or an organisation assisting a woman to have an abortion by booking her into a clinic or buying her a plane or boat ticket to England is guilty of an offence – because what the woman is intending to do is not illegal where she does it.

The Constitution and Abortion

What does our Constitution have to say about abortion? Unfortunately, nothing specific. Article 40, section 3, specifically guarantees to citizens the right to life, but is an unborn child a 'citizen'? Professor John Maurice Kelly considers not: he asserts that: 'presumably the attribution of citizenship to the foetus is *not* possible'.[30]

James O'Reilly, another constitutional lawyer, is more sanguine. He contends that:

> it would be but a little step for an Irish court to regard the life *in utero* as needing special protection, whether you want to regard this human life as a citizen or not. It is submitted that the protection that would be given to this life is such as to remove many of the fears expressed on abortion by critics of [*McGee*].[31]

Judge Walsh has gone very far in articulating a constitutional right to life for unborn children, but unfortunately the cases in which he did so did not raise the issue on their facts, so his statements do not constitute binding precedent for the future. In *McGee* v *Attorney General*,[32] Judge Walsh adverted to abortion in somewhat veiled terms when he said that:

> Any action on the part of either the husband and wife or of the State to limit family sizes by endangering or destroying human life must necessarily not only be an offence against the common good but also against the guaranteed personal rights of the human life in question.

He was much clearer on this question in *G.* v *An Bord Uchtala*,[33] when he said that

> [A child] has the right to life itself and the right to be guarded against all threats directed to its existence whether before or after birth. . . . The right to life necessarily implies the right to be born, the right to preserve and defend, and to have preserved and defended, that life. . . .

It should be stressed that Judge Walsh has been a lone voice on this subject. The other judges do not seem to be anxious to express any view on it until the issue is squarely raised in a case before them.

An alarming dimension to the problem is the experience in the United States, where, as we have seen, the Supreme Court relied on the concept of privacy (which developed from marital privacy) as a basis for making abortion available in effect on demand. Whether the Irish courts would follow the same analysis is far from clear. Certainly the importation of the concept of marital privacy in *McGee* in the majority, is a development that causes some concern. Academic analysis of the decision tends to doubt that there are implications regarding abortion. Mr James O'Reilly, for example, has gone so far as to assert that:

> Any commentator who seriously suggests that one can expect the Irish Supreme Court to arrive at a situation similar to [the American decisions] has not read the Irish Constitution [nor] the judgments in *McGee*, nor understands all the issues involved.

He describes those who predict such a possible development as 'prophets of doom'.[35] Similarly, Professor James Casey of U.C.D. has stated that:

> Those who argue that since the matrimonial privacy of *Griswold* v *Connecticut* led to the pro-abortion decision in *Roe* v *Wade*, the same must follow here from *McGee* v *A.G.* are guilty of an absurdly mechanical view of the judicial process.[36]

In my view, these commentators are guilty of too much vigour in ridiculing the possible developments in this country. No one seriously suggests that our Supreme Court would tomorrow recognise a constitutional right to abortion. Equally clearly, however, attitudes among the judiciary towards abortion may change in the coming years. If this happens, the introduction by *McGee* of the privacy concept into our jurisprudence may well serve to assist the constitutional case for abortion. Without such a concept, the constitutional argument in favour of abortion would be that much more difficult to establish.

It is noteworthy that in Mr O'Reilly's and Professor Casey's discussion of the subject, *both* commentators concede that the American decision of *Eisenstadt* v *Baird*[37] might be regarded as a relevant precedent in Ireland. In *Eisenstadt's* case the American Supreme Court at a stroke converted marital privacy into personal privacy.

Justice Brennan argued that a married couple was an 'association of two individuals each with a separate intellectual and emotional makeup' and accordingly that 'if the right of privacy means anything, it is the right of the *individual*, married or single, to be free from unwarranted Governmental intrusion into matters so fundamentally affecting a person as the decision whether to bear or beget a child.'

It is surely fair to comment that if this decision is to be regarded as a 'relevant precedent' in Ireland, those who are concerned about the implications for abortion may well be further alarmed. *Eisenstadt's* case set the course squarely for abortion, which was recognised only two years later in the United States in *Roe* v *Wade*.

Having said all this, may I stress again that I think that the likelihood of the right to abortion being recognised under our Constitution in the near future is extremely small. It seems much more likely that the rights of the unborn would be afforded constitutional protection and that the problem of citizenship would not present an insuperable hurdle to the Court. Since citizenship rights may be derived by inheritance, it would seem to be a strange denial of the realities to deny that these rights vest in an unborn child. Children in the womb derive wide-ranging property rights: it would be curious that they would nevertheless have no legal protection against termination of their right to life.

If the unborn child is to be afforded constitutional protection, it would, of course, be a futile protection if the only remedy he had was an action for damages which would go to the benefit of his estate. Obviously the remedy he would need would be of a more basic nature, namely one that would ensure his continued existence. An injunction prohibiting a proposed abortion would seem to be the most appropriate remedy. But may the Court grant an injunction to prevent the apprehended breach of a plaintiff's constitutional rights? It seems that it may. Professor John Maurice Kelly, in his recent treatise,[38] accepts that such proceedings would be possible.

Whether in specific cases an injunction would be effective is another matter. In England and America, courts have taken the view that it is impossible to prohibit an abortion in this fashion. Yet, if the consequences of defining an injunction were made absolutely clear to the defendant, this might have some effect. These consequences are indeed awesome. The defendant would be in contempt of court – for which commital to prison is the penalty; moreover an action for damages would also lie for destruction of the child's constitutional right to life.

One must be realistic here. A woman threatened with such sanctions could well decide to stay in England after her abortion rather than come back to prison in Ireland. Moreover, if such proceedings were to become frequent and well-known in our community, the effects might be entirely counterproductive – encouraging women to conceal their intentions from their spouses, boyfriends or families. In such circumstances, the chances of the woman being encouraged by persuasion not to have an abortion might be reduced significantly.

The Future

Let us look now to possible legislative developments in the future. What can be done by the law to protect the lives of the unborn? The question raises a number of problems, more in the political than in the strictly legal context.

The simple legal solution might appear to be on the following lines. If it is a criminal offence to have an abortion in *this* country, it may be argued that it should also be a criminal offence to have an abortion elsewhere. When the legislation was enacted in 1861, the laws in all European jurisdictions prohibited abortion (to a greater or lesser extent). There was therefore no need to make the offence extra-territorial since there was no possibility of evasion of the law by merely going to a neighbouring country. The laws in these neighbouring countries have now been changed so as to permit abortion in effect on demand. For *our* legislation now to provide that it should be illegal to have an abortion abroad would therefore *not* be changing what has since 1861 been the intended effect of our abortion law: on the contrary it would do no more than restore the position in the light of legislative developments elsewhere over which we have no control.

But would this legislation be desirable? It would be likely to be met with a barrage of criticism by those who favour abortion on the basis that it amounts to an inhumane attempt to persecute and make criminals of girls who have been driven by an uncaring society into taking this step as a last resort. It would be condemned as particularly unjust in the light of the limited access to contraception in this country.

Yet the philosophy on which these criticisms would be based can itself be challenged. If these criticisms have any validity, we should not only make it lawful to go to England to have an abortion: we should also have to make abortion lawful here. Yet the public policy of the State – and the virtual moral consensus in our society – opposes the legalisation of abortion. The view is taken that the life of the unborn child must be protected, however sympathetic one may feel towards the plight of the child's mother who is tempted to terminate its life. If we were to allow sympathy for the mother to stop us from regarding abortion as criminal when performed on an Irish girl in England, why should that sympathy stop at our shorelines? Similarly, if we regard abortion as wrong when performed here, why should it become right when performed fifty miles away?

If the law were to make it an offence to have an abortion in England, there would be a massive controversy: the proponents of the legislation would be vilified and branded as persecutors and hypocrites. It would require some strength of character for our politicians to withstand this barrage of criticism, but a strong argument can be made that our law should give such effect as it can to the principle that unborn life is entitled to be protected.

The practical difficulties of drafting such a law would, however, be enormous. The first problem would concern whom precisely the law whould cover? Obviously, it should not extend, for example, to an English woman residing in England who had a perfectly legal abortion there. If she came to Ireland for a visit some time later, she should scarcely be hauled off to Mountjoy for what she had done.

The position would scarcely be different where the woman was of Irish nationality but had lived almost all of her life out of Ireland. It would seem unjust that such a woman would effectively be exiled from Ireland if she were to have an abortion abroad.

It would seem that the law should be limited to persons with a close connection with Ireland at the time of the commission of the offence. Such persons could include those who are habitually resident here, or, more restrictively, Irish nationals who are habitually resident here.

Again, the legislation would be likely to be attacked on the basis that it 'discriminates' between different women – in this case on the basis that it discriminates against Irish women in favour of foreigners. This would not be a fair criticism but it would have strong emotive force.

The second principal objection against this type of legislation is that it would be virtually ineffective, and that legislation which does not work brings the whole legal system into disrepute. There is, of course, some general validity in this criticism, but, when the law is dealing with such an important matter as the protection of unborn life, this consideration should not be given too much weight.

Next, the law relating to abortion referral might be changed. Legislation could provide that it would be an offence to counsel, procure or assist in the commission of an abortion, whether in this country or abroad. There would be some problems in extending the scope of the criminal law to activities falling short of active procurement so as to cover what is called 'non-judgmental' advice and information. Clearly there are problems of definition here. If I say to a friend of mine who is pregnant: 'You know that abortions are readily available at a certain clinic in London or Liverpool for £90: the boat leaves every night at 10 p.m.', would I – or, indeed, *should* I – be guilty of a criminal offence? Is there any difference between *my* saying this and a counsellor in a family planning clinic?

The law could be so drafted as to attempt to distinguish between these cases but clearly much uncertainty and lack of clarity would be involved:

the legislation would be likely to be criticised by pro-abortionists on the basis that it denied free speech, and would be ridiculed as being unworkable in practice.

Perhaps the best course would be for the criminal law to go no further than provide that it would be an offence for a person to aid, abet or counsel an abortion whenever it is committed. This law would in many cases *not* go far enough to cover the cases where there at present is a real problem, but for it to attempt to do so would probably be counter-productive.

If the criminal law is not the best way to attack this problem, are there other legal methods? It seems to me that there are. In the United States, zoning laws and licensing systems have gone some way towards mitigating the damage done by anti-social activities, including abortion. The possibiity of creating a power to prohibit such practices by injunction, under sanction of heavy financial penalties, could also be investigated. The law relating to guardianship of children and wards of court could also be strengthened. What one does *not* want is the law making martyrs out of people, a number of whom are motivated by a strongly-held philosophy; what one *does* want is that they should be prevented from impeding the rights of the unborn of this country.

A more radical step might be contemplated in relation to the whole question of abortion. This would be to introduce a constitutional amendment guaranteeing in full terms the right to life of the unborn. Such a constitutional guarantee would not be strictly necessary in the sense that legislation protecting the unborn can be enacted under the existing constitutional provisions. Why, therefore, should such an amendment be contemplated?

I would see three possible interrelated benefits. *First*, it would have the effect of copperfastening the legal protection for unborn children. *Secondly*, the amendment would demonstrate a sincerity and strength of purpose regarding the protection of unborn life on the part of our people – who would, after all, be the authors of the amendment in voting for it at a national referendum. A favourable climate of public opinion in relation to the unborn might thus be established, rather than letting matters drift. *Thirdly*, the amendment would be a *positive* approach to the subject, stressing the policy of the protection of unborn life, which is the basis of the law in this area. [On 27 April 1981 the Pro-Life Amendment Campaign was launched in Dublin. In response to this two of the main political parties in the Republic, Fianna Fáil and Fine Gael, have given a commitment to propose a referendum on a Pro-Life Amendment to the Constitution. *Editor*].

There are, however, some important factors that should be taken into consideration before contemplating a constitutional amendment. *First*, it should be appreciated that such an amendment would give no continuing guarantee to the protection of unborn life. Like any other part of our Constitution such an amendment would itself be subject to repeal at anytime in the future when a majority of the voters wished to remove it. In the event of a gradual shift of public attitudes towards abortion, therefore, over the coming years, the enactment of a constitutional amendment now would prove to be only a passing protection.

Secondly, it might not be very desirable at present to raise unnecessarily the level of emotions on the subject of abortion by insisting on a national referendum on the subject. Unfortunately, the emotional aspects of abortion compete on more equal ground than do the philosophical and moral dimensions of the subject.

What one might find is that those who are pro-life would have brought on their heads a nasty emotive battle from which they might emerge with a less-than-impressive result, their cause having been constantly branded in public debate as anti-women, uncaring, doctrinaire and sectarian. The day when this battle may have to be fought may well come, but time is a strong argument against expediting it unnecessarily.

Sterilisation

The law relating to sterilisation[39] in this country does not appear to have been analysed by any court.[40] The uncertainty of the position must, therefore, be admitted at the outset. In this respect, this country does not differ from a number of others: it is only in very recent times that anything approaching a consensus regarding the legal position has been reached elsewhere. In the United States, the view was expressed in 1959 that 'the lawyer can do no more that offer an informed guess as to how the courts would regard a possible prosecution or damage suit, based on the performance of a contraceptive sterilisation'[41] and, even in 1966, the status under the criminal law of voluntary sterilisation was 'generally felt to be unclear'.[42] In England, the leading text book on criminal law stated in 1969 that 'the legality of the sterilisation operation is . . . not settled'.[43]

Therapeutic Sterilisation. One aspect of the subject does, however, seem to be reasonably clear. Therapeutic sterilisation seems to be without question lawful. The *boundaries* of therapeutic sterilisation may of course be a matter of disptue, but the principle seems clear.

Voluntary Sterilisation. It is voluntary sterilisation which gives rise to most of the legal uncertainty. Let us therefore look at specific aspects of this problem.

The Position at Criminal Law. It is an offence to inflict unlawful personal violence on another person.[44] This offence is generally referred to as assault or battery and, by legislation and at common law, a wide variety of acts are prohibited.

As a general principle, where the victim *consents* to the act, no offence is committed. There are, however, limits to the degree and nature of physical harm to which a person is permitted by the law to give an effective consent that will negative the criminal aspect of the act in question.[45] The problem is that, as Professors Smith and Hogan admit, 'where the line is to be drawn is by no means clear'.[46] At one extreme, it is clear that, for example, it would not be a defence to a charge of murder to claim that the victim asked to be killed.[47] At the other extreme, if a rugby player is accidentally bruised when he is being tackled, the tackler will not have committed an offence.[48]

So far, no court in this country has been called on to decide whether voluntary sterilisation is a criminal offence. Sterilisation appears to fall between the two extremes cited. The legality of the practice appears capable of challenge on two grounds, first that it involves a socially indefensible interference with the bodily integrity of the sterilised person, and secondly that it gives effect to a socially indefensible policy relating to family relationships and procreation. These challenges will be considered in turn.

It seems that a Court would be unlikely to consider sterilisation as criminal on the ground of interference with bodily integrity. However, it is quite open to a Court to hold that the act of sterilisation is *prima facie* a battery and that the desire of a person – particularly an unmarried person – to prevent pregnancy would not be sufficient justification for the act.

In England in 1954 the Court of Appeal considered this question in *Bravery* v *Bravery*.[49] There Lord Justice Denning expressed the view that when a sterilisation operation:

> is done with [a] man's consent for a just cause it is quite lawful – as, for instance, when it is done to prevent the transmission of an hereditary disease. But when it is done without just cause or excuse, it is unlawful even though the man consents to it. Take the case where a sterilisation operation is done so as to enable a man to have the pleasure of sexual intercourse, without shouldering the responsibilities attaching to it. The operation then is plainly injurious to the public intent. It is degrading to the man himself.
>
> It is injurious to his wife and to any woman he may marry, to say nothing of the way it opens to licentiousness, and, unlike contraception, it allows no room for a change of mind on either side. It is illegal, even though the man consents to it; for it comes within the principle stated by Stephen, J. (who was a great authority on criminal law) in *Regina* v *Coney*.[50] 'The principle as to consent seems to me to be this: When one person is indicted for inflicting personal injury upon another, the consent of the person who sustains the injury is no defence to the person who inflicts the injury, if the injury is of such a nature or is inflicted under such

circumstances that its infliction is injurious to the public as well as the person injured'.

That principle . . . clearly covers cases of sterilisation.[51]

The other members of the Court of Appeal in *Bravery* v *Bravery*[52] did not concur with Lord Justice Denning on this question (which they were not called upon there to decide) and expressly left the point open. Since 1954 the general view in England has shifted slowly but inexorably towards recognising the legality of voluntary sterilisation.[53]

Professors Smith and Hogan, the leading authorities on criminal law in England, state that:

> the infliction of any degree of bodily harm, however slight, is a battery unless [the victim] consents *and* the action can be positively justified by some rule of policy, such as that validating 'manly sports'. This leaves the law in an uncertain state and one depending very much on the views of the judges as to what is desirable, and what is undesirable, conduct.[54]

In favour of the view that voluntary sterilisation is 'desirable conduct' it might be argued that it is an efficient method of contraception which does not damage the physical or psychological health of the spouses. This issue must be resolved by reference to moral, medical and psychological considerations. The relative degree of importance to be attached to each of these factors obviously depends to some extent on the values of the particular court called on to determine the issue. After the decision of *McGee* v *A.G.*[55] it is difficult to envisage how the Court would hold that such an operation performed on a *married* person with the consent of his or her spouse for the purposes of contraception would constitute criminal conduct.[56] Where, however, the other spouse did not consent to the operation or where the person on whom the operation was performed was unmarried, it is far from certain that the Court would look with favour on the legality of the operation. Certainly, *McGee* does not go so far as to *require* the Court to make a holding one way or the other on this issue, but in its general philosophy it would seem to support the view that sterilisation performed on a spouse for contraceptive purposes at the wish of both spouses falls within the realm of marital privacy protected by the Constitution.

Artificial Insemination

Artificial insemination raises enormous legal problems. It is an area where some doctors have rushed in where wiser and more informed persons have not ventured.

There are, as you know, two principal types of artificial insemination – AIH[57] (where the husband is involved) and AID (where a third party, generally anonymous, is involved).

AIH does not pose very many legal difficulties. A child who is the product of AIH is legitimate. A difficulty arises, however, in the case of an AIH child, one of whose parents is impotent.[59] A marriage where one of the parties is impotent is voidable. The effect of a decree of annulment is that it retrospectively renders illegitimate the product of the union.[60] It would appear, therefore, that, in a case where an impotent spouse is concerned – and, it should be borne in mind, the spouse might be female[61] – AIH should not be contemplated without detailed legal advice in respect of such matters as the support, property and succession rights of the child who might be the product of this procedure.

The position of the AID child is far more complicated. The principal questions that arise are as follows:

(i) *Does the conduct of the wife constitute adultery?* The problem here for the law is how to adapt definitions relating to adultery to a scientific phenomenon – artificial insemination – which the judges in the past could not have anticipated.[62] The definitions of adultery that appear in the older decisions are therefore not conclusive, since the judges might quite easily have qualified them to some extent had they been able to take artificial insemination into account. The issue has never come before an Irish Court, but it is interesting to note that in other countries the courts have had great difficulty in coming to a satisfactory or consistent conclusion.

In a leading Canadian decision in 1921, the view was taken that the wife *did* commit adultery in such a case. In the view of Justice Orde:

> . . . the essence of the offence of adultery consists, not in the moral turpitude of the act of sexual intercourse, but in the voluntary surrender to another person of the reproductive powers or faculties of the guilty person; and any submission of these powers to the service or enjoyment of any persons other than the husband or the wife comes within the definition of 'adultery'.[63]

On the other hand, a Scottish decision[64] in 1958 has held that no adultery is committed in such a case. Lord Wheatley favoured the view that attention should be concentrated on the mutual surrender of both the sexual and the reproductive organs which normal sexual intercourse involved rather than on the procreative dimension.[65] In the United States the authorities are divided[66] but the general trend in academic analysis is in favour of the view that AID does *not* constitute adultery.[67]

It is impossible to predict how an Irish court would decide this issue, but there is a strong case for the view that it would hold that *no* adultery had been committed. Whatever moral opprobrium may attach to the 'voluntary surrender to another person of the reproductive powers or faculties of the guilty person',[68] and whatever the status of the child who is the product of that action, it would appear to strain unduly the well-established concept of adultery to extend it to the act of AID performed in clinical surroundings, with considerations of carnal pleasure totally absent.[69]

(ii) *Is there an element of cruelty?* The question whether AID constitutes cruelty[70] such as would entitle the other spouse to a decree for legal separation is somewhat easier to resolve than that of adultery since the concept of cruelty 'appears to be more ambiguous in meaning, more flexible, i.e. capable of expansion, than that of adultery'.[71]

It is submitted that, where AID is performed without the consent of the husband, such conduct should normally be regarded as cruelty, provided that the mental or physical health of the husband is affected.

Where, however, the husband consents to AID, he would be likely to be met by a successful defence of condonation or collusion.

(iii) *What is the legal status of a child conceived by AID?* The question of the status of the child conceived by AID would appear to be a more straightforward one but the position is hardly satisfactory as far as the child is concerned. It would appear incontrovertible that such a child (whether or not conceived with the consent of the husband) will be illegitimate.[72] The practical realities of the situation may well mean that the child's origins will never become publicly known and that the secret will die with the wife, husband and doctor. But the legal position, if the truth is ever disclosed,[73] would be as follows:

The child would have no succession rights against the husband's estate.[74]

He would have no right to be maintained by the husband, unless the husband were held by the Court to be *in loco parentis*[75] towards him or in a case where being aware of the child's origins, the husband 'has treated the child as a member of the family'.[76]

The donor would be capable of being sued for maintenance in relation to the child (assuming the unlikely fact that his identity was established) on the basis that he is the child's father.

AID and the Criminal Law

(i) *Falsification of Birth Records.* Turning now to the criminal law: it is an offence[77] to contravene any penal provision of the regulations under section 2 of the Vital Statistics and Births, Deaths and Marriages Registration Act 1952.[78] A person committing such an offence is liable to a fine not exceeding ten pounds.[79] The husband of a woman who conceives a child by AID would thus be guilty of an offence under this section, where he made a false statement that he was the father of the child.[80]

It is also possible that the husband or wife may be guilty of a common law misdemeanour akin to perjury where he or she is required to swear to the truth of any declaration that the child is the child of the husband's.[81]

(ii) *Conspiracy.* The husband and wife and the doctor who performed

AID could well fall foul of the criminal law of conspiracy. Halsbury states that: 'An agreement to commit a crime, whether that crime is punishable on indictment or on summary conviction, is an indictable conspiracy.'[82] The agreement between the parties to contravene the statutory regulations relating to the registration of the child's birth would appear to fall within this definition.

Moreover, it is a criminal conspiracy to agree to defraud another, or to commit a tort – that is, a civil wrong – which involves damage to another person, or to obstruct or prevent the course of justice.

It would appear that where a husband and wife agree to pass off a child conceived by AID as their legitimate child, they are necessarily thereby diminishing the property expectations of other persons. In some cases, of course, there may not be any person so affected, but in other cases there will be. Thus, for example, if the wife was already the mother of a child born out of wedlock, the birth of an apparently legitimate child would entirely defeat the succession entitlement of the child already born.[83] Property settlements may also exist, where provision is made for the eventuality of the birth of a legitimate child. In any of these types of case, the conduct of the husband and wife – and, it may be argued, in at least some cases, the doctor[84] – constitutes a conspiracy to defraud affected persons.

Why should the *doctor* be liable? The answer is that the object of the exercise is to produce a child which will be fraudulently passed off as the legitimate offspring of the husband and wife. The doctor may be fully aware of the specific facts which necessarily mean that the transaction in which he is participating will involve the commission of a wrong. He may, for example, be aware of the existence of a child whose legal rights will be affected by the fraud. It is more likely, however, that the doctor will be aware only in a general sense of the possibility of such persons existing. Whether a conviction against the doctor would be sustained in such a case is difficult to predict with any degree of confidence. The possibility of the doctor being convicted as aider and abettor of the conspiracy is also a real one.

Where the doctor performs AID on the wife *without* the knowledge of the husband, the position is far clearer. Both the doctor and the wife would appear to be guilty of conspiracy against the husband. Lord Denning has stated (extra-judicially):

> Secrecy and deception are the badge of conspiracy. If the wife and the doctor agree together to keep secret the fact that a child is illegitimate, they are guilty of a wicked conspiracy. If they do it without the knowledge or consent of the husband it is a gross fraud on the husband. He is made to maintain a child which is not his and which he is not liable by law to maintain. . . .[85] It is, I believe, if done without the knowledge or consent of the husband, a fraud and an unlawful, indictable conspiracy.[86]

It may also be argued that the doctor and the *donor* are guilty of a criminal conspiracy. Lord Denning has observed (again extra-judicially):

> What have they agreed? The whole essence of it is that it should be secret, not told to anyone. . . . And for what purpose? So that the donor should evade the responsibilities which by law attach to him. The natural and probable consequences of this is that he gets exception from maintenance or responsibility for his own child.[87]

Tort Law

Let us now consider what problems AID raises in tort law. Tort law is concerned with civil wrongs, such as negligence, defamation and trespass. AID has not yet been the subject of tort litigation in this country so the analysis of this aspect of the law must be regarded as somewhat hypothetical. Let us therefore consider the subject under different headings of liability.

(i) *Conspiracy.* It appears, that the mother, the donor and the doctor (as well as the husband, where he is a consenting party) may be guilty of conspiracy with respect to the financial interests of other persons which may be affected by their pretence that the child is the legitimate issue of the spouses concerned.[88]

(ii) *Fraud.* Where this conspiracy culminates in economic loss to any party, the conspirators may become liable for fraud.

(iii) *Negligence.* The doctor may be susceptible to an action for negligence, brought by the patient and her husband, based on failure to inform them of the likely consequences of the AID. The General Services Committee of the British Medical Association has warned that:

> The effect of AID on the patient and her husband must be considered carefully and the practitioner must exercise a proper degree of care and skill in ensuring that the patient and her husband fully understand the nature of the procedure and are given adequate warning of possible emotional troubles which might arise following the birth of a child. Should legal proceedings arise in circumstances where a couple are not capable of acquiring sufficient insight to cope with these problems it might be that a court would find a practitioner negligent in having failed to consider and deal with the possibility of these problems in advance.[89]

Whether it is negligent for the doctor to fail to warn the mother, her husband or the donor of the very important *legal* consequences following from AID is less certain. It would appear sensible practice for him to give such a warning.[90]

It is worthy of note that the Medical Defence Union in Britain recommends that the donor be required to sign a document acknowledging that it has been explained to him that the use of semen supplied might be held to be adultery and that he consents to supply semen on condition that his name is not disclosed and that the consent of the woman and her husband is obtained.[91]

Where the doctor is careless in his selection of a donor – as where the donor suffered from a serious physical or mental disability – he would appear to be guilty of negligence towards the woman and her husband.[92]

What constitutes due care might be difficult to determine in certain cases, since there is scarcely what could be called a customary practice on the matter in Ireland,[93] at all events not an overt one.

One basic point should, however, be noted. It is possible that the Court would dismiss an action based on negligence or the absence of informed consent because it regarded the whole practice of AID as being illegal and contrary to public policy.

What policy should the law take towards AID? It seems to me that it can take one of two possible courses – but no other. Either it makes the practice illegal and attempts to end the practice or it makes it legal and at the same time introduces very radical changes in family law. What cannot be done is to attempt to steer a middle course. This would ensure the maximum misery for all parties, putting a premium on fraud and suppression of the truth and on legal and logical inconsistency.

I personally would favour the first option, to end the practice of AID. I defer completely to those who have examined the medical and psychological aspects of the subject. From my reading of the materials as a non-medical person, I can only say that I am alarmed by what I have read and by what appears in at least some cases to be a willingness to embark on AID without a serious and detailed investigation of the particular circumstances of those seeking it and without sufficient empirical data on the success of the practice in the long term.

Conclusion

I said in my opening remarks that I would try to analyse the common legal philosophy running through the topics under discussion. It is difficult to see such a common philosophy unless one stands back from the details. If one does this, I think that it is possible to discern a development in many countries, particularly over the past decade, of the view that, in matters affecting procreation, individual autonomy and medical technology are to be allowed in combination to have precedence over any other moral or social norm. This is not a view that appeals to me. The danger of the destruction of far superior values is obvious – and, in the case of abortion, has already come to pass. The possibly less obvious, but no less important, dangers to family life and to society can also be identified.

I would prefer to see a different philosophy permeating these subjects – one which places a value on human rights, and which appreciates the true significance of the interpersonal and social dimensions of human conduct. The law can go some way towards keeping these values in focus: a concerned and caring medical profession can play a still more vital role.

10

Ethical Issues in Reproductive Medicine: from the Perspective of Moral Theology

MAURICE REIDY

Moral theology has to do with God and man. We take prenatal diagnosis, for example, and look at it from all the different angles. Why do it? Does it work? What are the risks? Is it legal? We then ask: Is it right? Being right goes deeper than the other questions. Even when something is done for a good motive, when it seems to work, when there is no great risk and it is legal – even then it might not be right. Ultimately if what we are doing is not right, the end is going to be tragedy. The only way that the answer to the question about being right can be arrived at is by seeing whether or not the thing is consistent with what God intends for us. And that is the business of moral theology.

According to the mind of Jesus, every person has eternal significance, every human creature is to be cared for and cherished, especially the one that is most in need. This is at the root of what God intends for us. For the moral theologian, particular difficulties will arise when questions are asked about how this caring is to be done, how far we should go in some instances, where we ought not to go in others. But the answers will come only when the difficulties themselves are seen from the standpoint of the basic insight which God has given. What does it mean to ask whether prenatal diagnosis is right? For the Christian the question becomes: is prenatal diagnosis a genuine form of care of mother and child?

In medical ethics the moral theologian continues to depend on the core message of Jesus, which informs and inspires the whole of the Christian ethic, and it is only by staying in touch with this message that he discovers a Christian response to the possibilities and ambiguities that present themselves in particular cases.

There are two broad and deeply interrelated areas of moral concern in reproductive medicine: human life and human sexuality. I propose to discuss each of these in turn, and to look at the particular questions that are associated with them in medical practice today.

Human Life

What value do we put on the human person, or on human life? To situate the question correctly, we should try to ask it in a context where there is likely to be widespread agreement about the answer; that is, we should pose the question in such a way that its general meaning will be easily realised, and the values that it seeks to elicit will be clear. What, then, is the value of a healthy male or female person, of between five and twenty-five years of age, who is in good standing with society? Or, what authority do we have in decisions that relate to the life and death of such a person?

Clearly, the concept of value, when applied to a person, refers to something that is intangible. One is not talking about economic value or 'willingness to agree' value. Persons can be unprofitable and ideologically uncooperative, yet they have value. Each person has a value that resides in himself because he exists. Each person has an identity and a right to exist which are vested in the person as person, an identity and a right which every other person is bound to recognise or concede, even if nothing is done to positively uphold or defend such identity and right.

Common agreement would suggest that each person who is healthy and who is between five and twenty-five years of age, and who is in good standing with society, is a subject in whom exists a proper identity and a proper right to exist by virtue of his or her own existence. Furthermore, common agreement would insist that we have no authority whatsoever to question the existence of such a person, or to put that life at any risk which was not for the medical good of such a person, presuming their consent, and that we have no authority whatsoever to end the life of such a person.

Now we should look at the variables in the question which are age, health, standing in society. Reproductive medicine encounters human life at what may paradoxically be called an 'advanced state of early age', it sometimes encounters human life in an acute stage of illness or handicap, and it sometimes encounters human life which enjoys a very questionable standing in the society in which it has been conceived. In what way is the answer to our basic question altered by these variables in a given subject? The value of human life is in no way altered by these circumstances, nor is there any alteration in our authority relating to decisions concerning life and death in such persons.

At this point, however, we begin to part company with common agreement, and this, I believe, by reason of three critical assumptions.

Three Assumptions

These assumptions are: first, that we have greater authority over the life of the unborn child than we do in relation to the child that is already born, or indeed, in relation to the adult; second, that human personhood does not come into existence until some time after the ovum has been fertilised; third, that it would be better for a handicapped foetus or infant not to live.

The first of these assumptions, that our authority over life in the womb is greater, is very deeply rooted in modern thinking. It has been reinforced by legal doctrines which assert that a mother has a right to decide whether or not she will continue with a pregnancy that has begun and that the unique state of natural dependency of a foetus becomes a ground for negating its moral status as an independent human being. When we are talking about life in the womb, the assumption runs, we are not talking about the right to life in the same sense as we mean it for life outside the womb.

As an illustration of this, I would cite the way in which direct abortion is often accepted as the lesser of two evils. A classic example of this acceptance is to be found in the book *Situation Ethics* by Joseph Fletcher. He tells of a doctor in a concentration camp who saved the lives of three thousand mothers by aborting them; the rule of the camp was that if a woman was pregnant she would be put to death. 'Even accepting the view that the embryos were "human lives" (which many of us do not), by "killing" three thousand the doctor saved three thousand and prevented the murder of *six thousand*'.[1]

The point I wish to make is that one aspect of this example, and one only, puts the defender of the basic right to life at a disadvantage. This aspect is not the concentration camp, it is the fact that the life in question is life in the womb. Suppose it had been decided that all able-bodied prisoners were needed for the war effort and in pursuance of this the order is given that every female prisoner who surrenders her children under seven years of age shall be transferred to a work camp; the children will be exterminated and the parents will be spared.

What is the substantial difference in this second example? Cannot the argument for the lesser of two evils be pursued equally well? Will not three thousand be saved? In the second example the emotional scales have been set at balance, there is a recognition that the lives at stake have an equal moral claim to survival. I want simply to show how modern assumptions about life in the womb carry an unexamined attitude to the value of life in the womb, to the right to life in the womb, and this attitude is patently false.

The second critical assumption, that human personhood does not come into existence until some time after the ovum has been fertilised, gives rise to an unfounded distinction in modern thinking whereby a difference is made between the right to life as it might apply at the blastocyst-embryo stage of human development, and the right to life as it might apply at the foetal stage of human development. There are no grounds in the scientific evidence that is to hand for drawing a moral distinction of this kind and no grounds for treating human life differently at any of these stages of development.

Speaking from strictly empirical premises, the geneticist Jerome Lejeune draws this pointed conclusion:

> I have never believed myself the ensoulment theories (whether theological or materialistic), pretending that the developing thing *in utero* will become a man some day, but it is not yet human before a given step has been reached. Indeed this 'given step' varies broadly from specialist to specialist. But that is not the question. What seems obvious to me, from all we know about genetics, is simply this: if a fertilized egg is not by itself a full human being, it never could become a man, because something would have to be added to it; and we know that does not happen.[2]

After fertilisation, a life has begun and no subsequent event, whether implantation or the division that leads to twins, or the commencement of the heart beat, or the beginning of electrical activity in the brain, substantially alters the progression of what is already present. In the case of identical twins there are two lives where formerly there was one; only in this sense do we know of a substantial alteration in twinning and it is a substantial addition rather than a substantial alteration. The phenomenon of identical twinning leaves intact the biological premise that human life has already begun.

It has been argued that many fertilised ova are lost in the very early days. But with our present knowledge, the fact of a percentage loss at this point is not itself an indication that human life is not present. Even if it could be conceded that fertilised ova that are spontaneously lost in the first few days are not human life, this would not permit us to conclude that all fertilised ova are not yet human life. What of those that are not lost, or which would not be if no steps were taken to interfere with their development? Furthermore, in many parts of the world, a great percentage of infants do not survive the first five years after birth, and yet no one would argue that this fact is an indication that they are not human.

The discussion concerning personhood in contemporary philosophy has given rise to a new consciousness of what it means to be a human person. In my view, however, it is misleading to expect at the present time that this discussion can lead to a satisfactory resolution of practical problems in medical ethics, where decisions have to be made about whether to do something which may have the effect of bringing life to an end. These problems occur not only in reproductive medicine but also in transplant surgery and in the management of patients on artificial life support systems. Practical decisions about life and death require practical criteria. For this reason I would argue that decisions concerning life and death ought to be made with the assistance of criteria for establishing whether death has taken place, rather than with criteria which would purport to indicate whether or not we are in the presence of a 'person'.

The critical question in this kind of situation is whether the patient is alive or dead, and if the patient is alive he is a full subject of appropriate medical and ethical concern. This applies also to life and death in the womb, at whatever stage of development. It is indeed difficult to *imagine* that a blastocyst is a human person; we are not required, however, to imagine this. The question is one of intellectual assent to the fact that a human life has begun, and that fact is incontrovertible. There is no ground for making an assumption that human personhood does not come into existence until some time after fertilisation.

The third critical assumption, that it would be better for a handicapped foetus or infant not to live, needs to be examined on a different plane. There may indeed be a truth in this. The question arises as to what practical decisions we are led to make in consideration of this truth. The assumption that death would be preferable to life may be based on a consideration of happiness after death, or on a subjective judgment that no life at all would be better for an infant who is severely handicapped. Each of these considerations may be present when decisions are made about elderly or terminally ill patients who are approaching death in great pain. Are not these considerations equally valid at or before birth?

I would argue that neither a religious belief in the after-life nor a subjective calculation of the value of a handicapped life is a sufficient basis for medical decision-making for other people without their consent. There is no obligation to prevent death when it is inevitable; it may be gladly, or sadly, accepted. Yet we are obliged to respect every life, and every human condition, and to cherish each person in an appropriate manner. The handicapped require great care, they have so much less than we do who are whole. Regret at handicap, and the fight to eliminate it, must not lead to a rejection of the handicapped person. This is not simply a charitable conclusion, but one of strict justice which recognises the proper claim of fellow human beings. A subjective judgment that a patient would be better off dead must never become a legitimising ground for the terminating of life or for the withholding of needed treatment.

Of these three critical assumptions, the first two, viz. that we have greater authority over life in the womb and that human personhood does not begin until some time after fertilisation, cannot be sustained at all, while the third, viz. that it would be better for the handicapped foetus or infant not to live, cannot be sustained as a sufficient guideline for making ethical decisions. As assumptions in medical ethics, the first two are false and all three are dangerous. Nonetheless, reflection on these three assumptions throws into greater relief the correctness of the three principles which I now propose.

1. The right to life applies at every stage of human development.
2. Human life begins at fertilisation.
3. The handicapped and the whole enjoy equality of rights and equality of consideration.

The first of these principles I take to be self evident: if there is such a thing as a right to life, then it must be possible to claim that right at any stage of human life. The second principle rests on the empirical evidence which verifies it. At the present time there is no evidence to suggest that human life begins at any time other than at fertilisation. The third principle, that the handicapped and the whole enjoy equality of rights and equality of consideration, must be conceded by every fair-minded person. To suggest that this principle is false is to overturn the whole ethical basis of our society.

Each of these principles underlies the treatment, which follows, of particular issues in reproductive medicine.

Induced Abortion

The first of the issues to be considered here is that of induced abortion, including abortifacient methods of birth control. In the medical world today there is a widespread acceptance of these practices. Even in medical textbooks 'termination' is the recommended treatment for several conditions. The consensus against abortion which runs through this book would not represent the general view.

In the light of the moral theory which I have presented it is evident that the practice of induced abortion, at whatever stage of pregnancy, and for whatever reason, must be considered gravely immoral. It runs directly counter to the medical presupposition of support for life. The unborn child, as well as the mother, makes an implicit claim on assistance, medical or otherwise, that the mother may seek. To directly terminate the life of the unborn is morally equivalent to the direct termination of any human life.

This same judgment applies to abortifacient birth control. Once it is recognised that human life begins at fertilisation then the moral significance of frustrating the progress of the fertilised ovum is obvious. Abortifacient measures, which depend on a sense of confusion regarding their mode of operation for their public acceptance, include the IUD. A recent report issued under the auspices of the Irish Medical Association concludes:

> The consensus of opinion at the present time is that the currently available I.U.Ds do not inhibit ovulation. While some effect on sperm transport may occur, especially with the medicated devices, the changes induced in the uterine milieu by the I.U.D. which prevent or interfere with the process of implantation of the blastocyst are considered to be the principal mode of action of the I.U.D.[3]

Nowadays oral contraception lays claim to a similar mode of action. Indeed 'contraception' is a misnomer, if conception is allowed to have possibly taken place. The original concept of 'the pill' involved the suppression of ovulation only, which prevented conception. Birth control by this method is now seen increasingly as a hazard to health. The modern 'pill' includes an abortifacient mode of action as one of the several effects which together promise to prevent the development of pregnancy, without harmful repercussions to health. This is not to say that a fertilised ovum is lost in each cycle; this may be the case, and it is the case if fertilisation occurs. In other words, the intention of very early abortion is part of the concept of modern birth prevention. For this reason it may be said that the whole idea of oral contraception has undergone a profound change in the last ten years.

Today, we have very grave problems in our society which are conducive to attitudes which encourage the seeking of abortion. It is at this level principally that the problem must be tackled. We need to set seriously about an alteration of some of our attitudes to new life, and this inevitably means we must encourage one another to be more questioning in regard to present assumptions about our own lives and their meaning. We need to encourage an openness to life, and a sense of welcome and hospitality towards the unborn, however embarrassing or world shattering their arrival may appear to be. Let small worlds be shattered, and let us take on earnestly the task of supporting parents where such support is needed. This demands from us an examination of education, values, relationships and traditional religious teaching to see in what ways those who seek abortion have arrived at their present position.

I suspect that there is much work to be done on the notion of 'responsible *fatherhood*' in our society, and not just in a moral sense, but in development of the whole notion of 'manness' in regard to male sexuality, both before and after marriage. Modern psychological theories of attachment and bonding confirm the basic insights of Christian sexual theory, and they remind us starkly that abortion is much more than a woman's problem. Behind the unwanting mother stands an unwanting father, and probably also the unwanting grandparents. I am not considering here the attitude of 'not wanting' a baby; what is at issue is the attitude we take up towards the 'unwanted' child and its mother when an unwanted pregnancy takes place.

The move to seek a constitutional amendment which would clearly recognise the right to life of the unborn is to be welcomed.[4] This must be part of a wide strategy that provides education and support and that looks beyond the shores of Ireland towards the establishment of similar recognitions in foreign jurisdictions, however daunting that task seems now.

Indirect Loss of the Foetus

The distinction between a direct and an indirect taking of life is well accepted in moral theology, although it is often misunderstood or misrepresented. In reproductive medicine this distinction is invoked when a womb which contains a foetus that is not yet viable has to be removed, and when a fallopian tube that will rupture is removed in an ectopic pregnancy. Each of these actions is good and necessary, the removal of a dangerously damaged and life-threatening part of the mother's body. A procedure which would countenance the loss of a foetus as an indirect consequence demands a careful and balanced diagnosis of mother and foetus, a diagnosis which would weigh honestly the sense of proportion, if any, regarding a possibility that the foetus might survive to viability and that the procedure could be deferred until then. This same principle applies to those difficult cases where a judgment must be made concerning treatment that may be necessary for the mother yet damaging to the foetus *in utero.*

Prenatal diagnosis

The important new developments of prenatal diagnosis bring with them a host of ethical problems. The procedures, considered in themselves, are quite moral, once due regard is taken of any inherent risk and the proportionate benefit of the procedure. As has been shown, prenatal diagnosis may offer opportunities for important medical developments in support of life. However, another aspect of the reality of the situation is that in many countries these procedures and abortion go hand in hand. Indeed it may be said that amniocentesis and abortion are coming to be synonymous terms in the public mind. This represents a complete distortion of prenatal diagnosis and creates a problem for the doctor who is asked to provide it. The request for prenatal diagnosis cannot be detached from the interest of the foetus, and the doctor's response to this request, whether in carrying out the procedure, or in communicating the information that the procedure yields, cannot be detached from the likely consequences of that response.

With the availability of reliable prenatal diagnosis there would seem to be a growing acceptance among doctors today of the *selective abortion* of the very severely handicapped. It is argued that the severely handicapped foetus may not live very long and that it will be a heavy burden on its parents and family. In the course of this book several very distressing kinds of condition are mentioned.

In the literature of medical ethics this issue is frequently argued in terms of 'quality of life'. This concept however, is not a suitable one for ethical decision-making in this area. There seems to be a frighteningly easy transition from discourse about quality of life to discourse about 'who shall live and who shall die'. Decision-making will be better served by reference to the inalienable rights of any human subject, handicapped or otherwise, to equality of consideration and appropriate care. This point is put forcefully in a wide ranging and thoughtful article by the ethicist Karen A. Lebacz:

Even more than abortion on demand, it seems to me, selective abortion

> embodies principles of unequal treatment which violate fundamental moral and legal equality of all human beings. In the long run, this violation of fundamental rights of equal treatment is a more serious threat to the 'quality of life' of all of us than the birth of numerous children with defects will ever be. I am heartened by the seriousness with which this matter has been taken in general both by parents and by physicians, nonetheless it is a dangerous move to aid parents by eliminating their children. We must beware of the implications of moving to a 'quality of life' ethic in which persons are judged according to their social utility and hence 'some are more equal than others'.[5]

It is evident that in medical ethics action and attitude go together, they depend on one another and they interact upon one another. One has only to look at the evidence that shows how ready society is to eliminate the handicapped members before birth, to realise that the modern attitude towards handicap is highly questionable. The ethicist Leon Kass makes this telling observation:

> It is ironic that we should acquire the power to detect and eliminate the genetically unequal at a time when we have finally succeeded in removing much of the stigma and disgrace attached to victims of congenital illness, in providing them with improved care and support, and in preventing, by means of education, feelings of guilt on the part of their parents.[6]

With these points in mind I would argue that there is no place for selective abortion in medical practice. There ought to be no exceptions to this general rule. In support of this view, I would like to consider in some detail the difficult, and conscientiously disputed, case of anencephaly.

The anencephalic foetus has no brain and it will die at birth. Many doctors who are strongly opposed to abortion would consider that this case constitutes a general exception. As a moral theologian I do not wish to engage in what might appear to be a black and white confrontation on this point. I wish simply to state what I perceive to be reasonable considerations which support a moral prohibition on the direct taking of all innocent life even in the most extreme case of handicap. While anencephaly will not occasion the kind of hardship that may come with a severely handicapped child that will survive birth and live on for some years, yet the very nature of this handicap seems to raise very pressing questions both for the moral argument which I have outlined, and for the practical counselling of parents whose child has been diagnosed as being in this condition.

The following seven points describe the anencephalic condition as it is perceived medically:

1. The anencephalic foetus is the fruit of human conception.
2. It fulfils the criteria of being a foetus, although it has no brain.

3. It is alive, not dead.
4. The majority of these would cause no harm to the mother.
5. Anencephaly is a condition which is never likely to be remediable.
6. Many will die during labour and the remainder will die shortly after delivery because they lack lower brain function.
7. The facilities for diagnosis of this condition are likely to improve considerably, so that certain diagnosis would be available by twelve weeks gestation.

There are those who would argue that the most pressing question turns on whether the anencephalic foetus is human. As we have noted, it is the fruit of human conception and it fulfils the criteria of being a foetus, although it has no brain. In my view the philosophical debate concerning the nature of personhood has not reached the kind of maturity as yet which would allow us to conclude with moral certainty that the anencephalic is not a human person. In addition, more needs to be known about the cause of this condition.

I would argue that the most pressing question turns on what is meant by saying that the foetus is alive. Since the advent of 'brain death', the point is made that the anencephalic is 'brain dead', and that the mother may be considered as a 'life support system' that simply keeps basic functions going. The foetus is compared to a corpse on a machine, the ventilation and circulation of which is being maintained. I think that one has to concede the brain death argument – there is no brain at all. Yet I think one may question whether there is any right to remove the foetus, pre-term, on the basis that it is on 'artificial life support'. Brain death is not absolute; it becomes a final criterion that death has taken place when accompanied by the spontaneous cessation of heart and lungs. 'Brain death' and 'death' are not necessarily the same thing.[7] For these reasons I would tend to argue that the abortion of an anencephalic foetus is the abortion of a foetus that may be presumed to be human, and not yet dead.

In addition to the question of brain death, the point is made that this foetus can never be viable. Lack of viability however does not make it absolutely exceptional. There are several conditions in which foetuses will never be viable. Examples of this situation are Potter's syndrome, where the baby has no kidneys and will die once removed from the mother's body, and advanced Rhesus incompatibility, where a foetus will die at term because of haemolytic anaemia. To make non-viability a ground for abortion would certainly be an admission of the direct taking of life that we know to be human.

Non-treatment of severe congenital malformation

And so we come to discuss the difficult issue of selection for treatment or non-treatment of defective newborn infants. The issues which present themselves here are not at all as clear cut as those which arise in abortion. They are further complicated by developments in medical technology which have made it possible for many more of the handicapped to become survivors than was previously the case. One has to ask whether such developments are always to the advantage of a handicapped child.

There are two related strands to the moral discussion: What are our values? What specific things do these values incline us to do or not to do? Our task is to discover that coalescence of value and action which will enable us to make right judgments of conscience in the best medical interest of these vulnerable patients. The following observations may be made as a beginning:

1. The obligation to prolong human life is not unlimited.
2. The acceptance of death can be a perfectly moral response in some circumstances.

Much of the debate on selection has focused on objective medical criteria which have been put forward to facilitate decision-making in cases where infants have spina bifida.[8] This concept of selection raises the following serious difficulties:

1. It recognises that some infants will go without treatment who would in fact benefit from it, i.e. they will suffer directly from the decision not to treat and they will survive in a worse condition than if they had been treated.
2. It requires that the person making the selection comes to a decision that the infant would be better off were it to die, so that treatment may be withheld, and the sequelae of non-treatment be allowed to take place, even though there may be no clear indication that the child will soon die.
3. It further requires that the sequelae of non-treatment be not treated, as this would only defeat the whole purpose of the original decision, bring further hardship to the infant, and this requirement seems to demand some kind of intention that the infant should die, on the part of those responsible for its care.

Having mentioned these difficulties, I would not want to argue that every infant should be selected for maximum treatment. How then is one to balance the conflicting values that may present themselves in some cases of severe handicap, when it is not clear that available treatment is to the advantage of the infant, and how is one to help parents and nurses to gain some insight into decisions in which they will be participating, and into the regime of subsequent treatment or care which decision not to treat will certainly involve?[9]

I would suggest that the problem be seen as one of appropriate care, and not primarily as one of selection or non-selection based on criteria which, at least when applied to some cases, admit to being arbitrary. Every infant is due appropriate care. This can be made more specific by insisting that every infant is due the ordinary means of care, treatment and nourishment that are occasioned by its present condition. In general, ordinary means are those which:

1. promise recovery, either from present condition or illness, or from general grave condition associated with handicap;
2. do not place great burden on patient with no realistic hope of good prognosis;
3. satisfy conscience of doctor that this is normal and reasonable intervention to prevent or correct this condition in any patient.

The purpose of the distinction between ordinary and extraordinary means is to help us decide whether a treatment is morally of obligation. We are obliged to take or provide ordinary means; we are not obliged to take or provide means that can be considered extraordinary in a particular case. Extraordinary means would be those which are unduly hazardous, experimental, or which place a great burden on the patient. Means which would place an undue burden on the patient would be those that occupy the patient to such an extent and with such hardship that his survival will always continue to be bound up with the painful struggle necessitated by the means themselves, when there is no prospect of the means being able to provide or restore any capacity for human living. Admittedly, it would seem to be inevitable that some kind of subjective judgment concerning 'quality of life' will enter into decision-making at this point. Notice, however, that I have laid the emphasis on the unacceptability of the means available. There can be no suggestion of unacceptability regarding the handicapped person, no matter how distressing the condition may be.

This application of the moral distinction between ordinary and extraordinary means to cases of spina bifida is presented in greater detail by the moral theologian Warren Reich in his article 'Quality of Life and Defective Newborn Children; an Ethical Analysis'. Admittedly, in the end, the decisions that have to be taken are subjective decisions based on the assessments of those responsible:

> This obviously calls for a 'subjective' judgment about the reasonable limits of hardship; but so do the majority of judgments of 'extraordinary means' – whether in the 'old' medical ethics or the ethics of the 'new medicine'. The real question here is whether anyone is entitled to make a proxy judgment relative to the treatment of another incompetent person (for such judgment always entails a value component). The author believes such a judgment can and must be made and that abuses will only be avoided or minimised by a complex set of considerations, including a totally serious commitment to the general rule of sustaining human life and to the reasons (human dignity and human fidelity) that underlie it, the refusal to subordinate adverse medical criteria to utilitarian or merely consequentialist considerations, and a dedication to alleviating suffering coupled with the conviction that a life with handicap and suffering can be meaningful. This framework

for medical decision-making cannot easily be codified – certainly no more so than the formulas for any value-laden art of human behaviour. Yet this approach is preferable to a medicoethical system that would categorically and systematically exclude as beneficiaries of a duty to sustain human life those infants or groups of infants who lack some specific asset or some relative endowment.[10]

In this debate today increasing reference is made to the social circumstances of relatives and to the amounts that society may be asked to pay for the maintenance, or assisted maintenance, of handicapped children. This ought not to divert us from the fact that appropriate care is basically a patient-centred issue. In line with my basic moral approach, I would have to argue that the ethical issues that arise in the care of a handicapped foetus or infant are to be resolved in the same way as for any handicapped or injured person, of whatever age.[11]

In this light too, the relevance of social indices is to be assessed, with the clear knowledge that we presume the consent of the person concerned for whatever we judge to be appropriate. If social indices are likely to have a bearing on what we might consider to be appropriate for a seriously injured twenty-five year old, whose consent we presume, then and only then can they be said to have relevance in our care of an infant. At the very least, I would consider this to be highly problematic, unless it could be shown that the particular social indices had such a bearing on the medical prognosis that this in turn was gravely affected. In our society, which provides a form of socialised medicine, the argument which would turn on social circumstances would seem to be very questionable, and I would argue in favour of being bound only by the particular medical indication, and the presumption of consent for whatever would be medically indicated in what would be considered normal social circumstances of time and place.

Human Sexuality

We come now to the other theoretical area implicit in the ethics of reproductive medicine, where two questions arise: What is the human meaning of reproduction, and, what is the human meaning of sex? Some examination of these questions is necessary in order to understand the moral issues that underlie attempts that may be made to assist the infertile couple to have their own child, and the moral issues involved in the control of fertility and the avoidance of conception.

The human meaning of reproduction centres on a man and a woman who wish to be parents and who have some kind of personal and procreative bond between them which would make them suitable for that task. When we are speaking of sperm and ovum, we are speaking not only of a possible blastocyst and embryo, but of a possible foetus and child and adult. When we speak of a female who produces an ovum, we are speaking of a person who is a subject of maternal instincts, responses and wishes. When we speak of a male who produces sperm, we are speaking of a person who is a subject of paternal instincts, responses and wishes.

Are such persons concerned to see the life that they conceive through its various dependency stages until adulthood? And are they concerned about the continuing interaction between themselves as spouses and parents which provides the optimum and proper human context for themselves and for their children at each stage in life? There is much more common agreement than we might suppose in the expectations of men and women in these matters, at least at the level of ideals. A good relationship and a good family prospect are the indispensable starting points for a moral theory of human reproduction. The human meaning of reproduction refers to the coming to be of a new person, and that development cannot be abstracted from the reality of that person's father and mother.

Human meaning refers also to the actual processes of reproduction. Until the modern era very little was known of these processes. The act of intercourse is the object of special reverence in Christian perception because that act participates in the mysterious dispositions of divine providence whereby new life is engendered. This participation is the origin of the term 'procreation'. A more exact knowledge of the human processes, both physical and psychological, makes possible a more balanced appraisal of moral questions in these areas.

The advancement of what is called scientific knowledge has been accompanied by alterations of philosophical emphasis. The most important of these alterations may be designated by the word 'personalist'. This word is not easy to define, but it represents a move away from 'physical nature' considered in itself, and a move towards the 'personal', 'relational', 'human meaning' aspects of the experience of human nature. These emphases have had an important influence on the articulation of Church teaching. They make their first appearance in the encyclical letter *Casti Connubii* of Pius XI (1931), which was a comprehensive presentation of Catholic teaching on marriage; they appear more insistently in the teaching of Pius XII, (1939–1958) and they may be said to have been 'canonised' in the Second Vatican Council (1963–1965), particularly in the document *Gaudium et Spes*. These developments play an important role in the working out of the moral issues that will now be considered.

Assisting Human Reproduction

Under this heading a host of questions present themselves, many of them seeming to spring from the pages of science fiction. Artificial insemination and *in vitro* fertilisation are being accepted today as legitimate approaches to the making of human beings. In order to focus clearly on the moral aspects of these procedures, it is necessary to keep before our eyes the simple human model of the family. The family is the key to the morality of reproduction.

At the heart of the human family is the couple. The man and woman unite in the sexual act through which life is conceived. This momentum is natural and it is personal. A child is born, not simply in response to parental desire, but as a gift of God who is the Creator. The coming to be of a human being is not a secular or a scientific matter, it touches on the sacred ground of divine providence and human dignity.

The critical moral question is this: to what extent may technology be permitted to supersede natural processes which are defective, when no threat is implied either to human life or to the proper human relationships and actions within and through which human life is to be conceived. At the conceptual level, theology is quite open to an understanding of life and human nature that is assisted by inventiveness and technology.[12] We have nothing to fear from research that is respectful of the human person.

Artificial insemination by donor is not respectful of the human person. Children are born whose fathers are numbers on a file. This procedure bypasses both the act of intercourse and the natural context of father and mother. The donor begets without ever knowing the child that will be conceived of him, or its mother. This contradicts the whole notion of parental responsibility and the bonding that should take place between father, mother and child.

A person does not have a 'right to a child' as such. Spouses confer on one another a right to intercourse together, by which means a child may be born to them. It is immoral for a wife to seek a child by another man. It is equally wrong for a husband to seek a child by another woman.

In the earlier part of this century theologians were somewhat open to the idea of AIH, that is, artificial insemination by a husband.[13] However, the teaching of the Church, as expressed by Pope Pius XII, is opposed to this practice, although it admits 'the use of certain artificial means of facilitating the natural act or of helping its fulfilment when normally carried out'.[14]

Theologians continue to discuss the arguments concerning AIH. There would be a strong awareness today of the way in which procreation unites a couple. The gift of a child complements the bond of husband and wife, and furthermore, it complements for them the unitive meaning of their sexual encounter. The gift of a child is an affirmation of the parents and it is an affirmation of the meaning of the act of intercourse 'when normally carried out'. This is part of a more modern perception in which marriage is defined in terms of two essential and complementary 'ends', the 'unitive' and the 'procreative'.

In particular, theologians are asking whether, in the light of personalist influence, acts that are associated with AIH could be considered to be unitive and procreative, as is the act of intercourse.[15] Could AIH be considered to be relational, unitive and procreative, being done for the purpose of expressing conjugal unity and giving new life? The final judgment on the validity of these considerations remains with the teaching authority of the Church.

This same question may be asked concerning *in vitro* fertilisation. While technological developments of this kind would appear at first to be contrary to the Christian approach to procreation, there are other important considerations which weigh in their favour. It may soon be possible, for example, to create the conditions for the whole gestation of a human being outside the womb. If this technology were to offer the possibility of survival to a very early foetus that was known to be under immediate threat (e.g. the removal of a cancerous uterus, the loss of an embryo in the rupture of the fallopian tube in an ectopic pregnancy), then it would be very difficult to condemn it. In the years ahead we may expect that moral theology will continue to give these problems the serious and sympathetic consideration which they deserve.

On the other hand, should the process of *in vitro* fertilisation involve the intentional discarding of fertilised ova at the blastocyst stage, or at any stage, then this is a discarding of life that must be presumed to be human, and it is therefore gravely immoral. Similarly, the practice of freezing the blastocyst with a view to inserting it in the womb at a later stage would seem to show an incredible disregard and lack of respect for human dignity and human rights.

Family Planning

We come now to the other side of the coin, the avoidance of pregnancy, and family planning. In this matter there are indications of revolution in the perceptions of theology. The controversy in the Church concerning artificial birth control has created an unintended smokescreen which has hidden from view some major alterations of perspective. As we have seen, the perspective in which childbearing was seen as the main moral justification for sexual activity, and indeed for the existence of human sexuality, is no longer tenable in the way in which these matters were perceived in the past. Admittedly, the 'mutual comforting of husband and wife' did occupy a secondary place in earlier theology, but it was not one of major spiritual significance. Sexual activity is seen today as a proper dimension of human expression and experience whereby a couple relate to one another as man and woman, and as father and mother.

In theological and spiritual writing today there is a renewed appreciation of human sexuality. The foundations of this have been described in the doctrinal teaching of the Second Vatican Council's *Gaudium et Spes*, in the encyclical letter *Humane Vitae* of Pope Paul VI, and in the recent apostolic exhortation regarding the role of the Christian family in the modern world, *Familiaris Consortio*, of Pope John Paul II. These foundations consist in the mutually complementary ends of marriage as unitive and procreative. The essential unitive dimension of human sexuality links in with the whcle new secular awareness of sexuality in this century, particularly evident in psychology and serious literature, and with the new trends in theology which tend to invest human life on earth with a renewed sense of dignity and vocation, deriving from our perceptions of God's creation of the world, and his incarnation in human history.

These emphases are not without their own human difficulties. In the society in which we live, a lot of disillusionment is expressed concerning sexuality, marriage and spirituality. It is argued that the ideals of life-long commitment are no longer possible, that they were appropriate to a former age but not to the modern time with its pressures for change and personal development. It is argued that the reality of marital breakdown and of divorce make traditional moral discourse unrealistic and out of touch.

There is a danger that human sexuality will be invested with expectations of fulfilment that it is unable to sustain and not just human sexuality but human companionship and friendship. Indeed, there are those who would say that at the present time sex is being asked to bear a responsibility for the making and maintenance of human happiness which it cannot, was never able, and was never intended, to bear. Without a sense of realism and true religion the human condition is in danger of being built up with a greater weight of expectation than many people can hope to realise. We live in an imperfect world, and we live with one another's imperfections. These are an inevitable dimension of the milieu of human life and human love.

It would seem that one of the crisis points in the Catholic understanding of these matters has been occasioned by the realisation that sexual intercourse is for the most part not procreative. On most occasions when the act is performed there is not an intention to conceive, indeed it is most likely that the intention is not to conceive. For this reason we urgently need to explore the unitive side of our definition. Traditional Catholic thinking, since the early centuries, has defined marriage in terms of 'the bond', 'the children', 'the sacrament'. The emphasis in the more recent past has been frankly procreative, and our spiritual and theological heritage is not well equipped for the adjustments that now face us. What follows is an attempt to sketch out the kind of ground within which these adjustments will be made.

Sexual experience is perceived as having strong and deep links with human personality and with human needs. It has, moreover, strong and deep links with the reciprocity of life together of husband and wife. Sexual experience, and especially the experience of sexual intercourse, cannot be separated from happiness, from anxiety, from emotional tension, when these are present. It cannot be separated from the need to love, and to be loved, in the body. But if the meaning of sexual encounter is to be sought at the level of good sexual intercourse, then all of those factors are relevant which bear on good personal union. A moral theory of sexuality, therefore, must understand sexual intercourse in terms of what is possible and desirable both procreatively and unitively. Intercourse is, or ought to be, a unifying act of a man and woman who seek the most open and total way in which they can hold one another and entrust themselves to one another.

Sexual union is physical, it is personal and it is spiritual. It is the awareness of this whole reality which makes sexual satisfaction so essentially interpersonal, and indeed it is the lack of the whole reality which makes a difficult marriage so deeply painful. The good union is one in which there is a community of body and spirit. This idea of union or 'communion' between a man and a woman is central, and the normal and complete experience of this union takes place in the state of marriage. In marriage a man and a woman live together with the expectation of being husband and wife to one another, and of being parents to the children they may have. A merely physical basis for sexual moral theory is not sufficient; human nature is spiritual, and human sexuality is part of a man and a woman's spiritual nature. The Bible reminds us that in the perspective of God, man is seen as a human couple:

> God created man in his own image; in the image of God he created him; male and female he created them (*Genesis* 1:27).

Jesus and Marriage

I would like to refer here to the teaching of Jesus on marriage. In this passage he is asked to comment on the grounds for divorce in Israel, a subject which was hotly contested by two schools in his day, one of which admitted narrow grounds for divorce; the other admitted very wide grounds. In giving his answer, Jesus goes back behind the question to state what marriage really is:

> Some Pharisees approached him, and to test him, they said. 'Is it against the Law for a man to divorce his wife on any pretext whatever?' He answered, 'Have you not read that the Creator from the beginning made them male and female and that he said: This is why a man must leave his father and mother, and cling to his wife, and the two become one body? They are no longer two, therefore, but one body. So then what God has united, man must not divide'. (Matthew 19: 3–6).

We are used to looking at these words through spectacles which are labelled 'divorce'. Let us remove those spectacles for a moment and look directly at what Jesus is saying about marriage. Much of what he says is quoted from the first two chapters of the book of Genesis, which tell the story of Adam and Eve in the Garden of Eden. We find that Jesus is in touch with the deeper issue underlying the original question. His perception is that man and woman become one, and that they are brought together by God. Note the simple sequence of ideas: male and female, the two become one body, what God has united. The uniting intention of God is not to be understood in a legal sense only, any more than the reality of marriage is only legal. It is the intention of the Creator that male and female are for one another, and more than this, the Creater is in some sense present in and party to the bond that a man and woman make together.

He is present in the union, and in the way in which it is experienced, in good times and in bad, and we believe that he is present in the procreation that takes place when a child is conceived. The fact that due to human insensitivity and sinfulness the circumstances of conception are sometimes tragic and brutal ought not to blind us to the mysterious creative event which is the beginning of new life.

This teaching of Jesus, with its showing of God in the marital bond, needs to be related to sexual theory. The bond is of its nature a sexual bond, and one that is nourished and nurtured by sexual loving. The making of this bond between a man and a woman is a practical thing, and it is done in practical ways through affirmation of the person and time spent attentively together. This affirmation and attention contains a pleasurable sexual dimension, the disappearance of which is a cause for anxiety and lack of confidence in the relationship.

It can happen in discussion of the spiritual aspects of life that an abstraction takes place which divides soul from body. The spiritual domain is presumed to be the domain of the separated soul. This kind of abstraction is a grave mistake. Soul and body belong together as different aspects of the human person. Indeed body and sense are the intimate bearers of the soul. In the human encounter, it is at the bodily and sensual and emotional levels that the bruises and barriers of the soul are often most keenly felt. Put positively, it is at these human levels that the true communion of souls in marriage is properly acknowledged and affirmed.

Moral Theory

A moral theory of sexuality is related to an attitude that seeks intercourse on those occasions when there can be complete openness of body and spirit. There will be occasions when intercourse is sought in the fertile time, occasions when it is sought in the infertile time, and occasions when it is sought regardless of fertility, and consciously so. Within this kind of openness and control intercourse is a consummation of the whole person, the whole love, the whole pleasure. The suppression of anything basic that is present, whether of the heart or of the loins, is a suppression of part of the self and therefore of part of the union.

In a word, a moral theory of sexuality comprehends the whole relationship of a man and a woman and God, and asserts the moral goodness of sexual acts which recognise the realities of unity and procreation that are present at any moment, whether in happiness or anxiety, whether it is intended to conceive or not to conceive. This is the pivotal point about the openness of marriage between persons, and its challenge at every human level, sexual and otherwise. This is the point of insight or vision, which because of its 'ideal' quality, becomes the point of reference for a moral theory of human sexuality. Such a theory would seek to give guidance to all couples in their quest for the good. It may be asked from the point of view of moral theology whether it would be desirable that couples should experience one another sexually as I have described, and I suspect that common agreement would say 'yes', at least at the level of theory. Getting the theory right is essential; what is humanly desirable is a most reliable indication of what is moral.

Responsible Parenthood

Having made these points, let us look now at family planning. There are two levels to this, a theoretical one and a practical one. At the theoretical level a major theme is that of responsible parenthood.[16] Apart from a general recognition that responsible parenthood would take into account the true unitive needs of husband and wife as well as the true human needs of existing and anticipated children, and the needs of church and society, there has not been any detailed attempt to develop the concept in a way which would be of assistance to couples. Just to take the negative aspect, because that is the one that naturally tends to dominate in these pages, there is very little guidance in moral theology on those difficult situations when a couple together, or one partner alone, must decide that the proper moral conditions for conception are not present, whether those conditions reside in the state of the marriage and family in question, or in the health or lack of it in the procreative faculty of the parents. This is where genetic indications may be important, for example, or any pathological contra-indication to pregnancy which may exist in the mother. The small print of the concept of responsible parenthood needs to be spelled out by moral theology at the present time.

Humanae Vitae (1968)

At the practical level, the issue in family planning is the proper means. This became the dominant question in the 1960s, leading to the encyclical letter *Humanae Vitae* of Pope Paul VI. At the Synod of Bishops in Rome in 1980 this encyclical was once again endorsed, along with the teaching of the Second Vatican Council's teaching on marriage, as having spoken 'prophetically to our times, clearly affirming the Church's ancient but ever new teaching on marriage and the transmission of human life'.[17] *Humanae Vitae* is clearly a prophetic document which affirms the human and procreative dimensions of sexuality in a language and perspective particularly apt to our age. The decline of sexual morality and of respect for unborn life in recent decades is a stark witness to the consequences of sundering these two essential dimensions of human sexuality. This is not to deny the difficulties that many have experienced with the moral teaching of the encyclical. I believe that these difficulties will be overcome only when we have seized wholeheartedly the full moral insight which *Humanae Vitae* proclaims, and remembering that contraception is always a disorder, we undertake the task of relating this to those other important moral principles which offer guidance in situations of genuine perplexity.

There are three related aspects in the teaching of this document:

1. The doctrinal aspect, in which the unitive and procreative dimensions of marriage and sexuality are affirmed, and declared to be indispensable to one another (*H.V.* 12).
2. The moral aspect, whereby any use of the sexual act in which there is either neglect of the unitive dimension, or supression of the procreative dimension that is present, is excluded (*H.V.* 13, 14).
3. The pastoral aspect, in which it is recognised that many couples will find this teaching difficult and that therefore a pastoral policy which aims at promoting the ideal, even when this ideal is not being achieved, is the one to be followed with each couple. This is why couples are exhorted to continue to frequent the sacraments of the Eucharist and of Penance (*H.V.* 19, 20, 25, 27).

In the controversy which followed *Humanae Vitae*, this pastoral dimension has frequently been forgotten.

Familiaris Consortio (1981)

Pope John Paul II is the author of this document which is the most recent expression of magisterial teaching on the whole subject of marriage in the modern world. The question of family planning receives detailed consideration. The themes of *Humanae Vitae* are explored with a personalist and philosophical emphasis which are characteristic of the present Holy Father. I have chosen to present here two quotations concerning the meaning of human sexuality and the moral progress of married people. I realise that it is difficult to make a selection from a whole text which is itself wide-ranging and profound, nevertheless these two illustrations will give an impression of the Church's position on these matters today.

The first quotation refers to contraception and the meaning of human sexuality, and it concludes with an in-depth description of the bodily and spiritual conversation or dialogue between man and woman:

When couples, by means of recourse to contraception, separate those two meanings that God the Creator has inscribed in the being of man and woman and in the dynamism of their sexual communion, they act as 'arbiters' of the divine plan and they 'manipulate' and degrade human sexuality – and with it themselves and their married partner – by altering its value of 'total' self-giving. Thus the innate language that expresses the total reciprocal self-giving of husband and wife is overlaid, through contraception, by an objectively contradictory language, namely, that of not giving oneself totally to the other. This leads not only to a positive refusal to be open to life but also to a falsification of the inner truth of conjugal love, which is called upon to give itself in personal totality. . . . The choice of natural rhythms involves accepting the cycle of the person, that is the woman, and thereby accepting dialogue, reciprocal respect, shared responsibility and self-control. To accept the cycle and to enter into dialogue means to recognise both the spiritual and corporal character of conjugal communion, and to live personal love with its requirement of fidelity. In this context the couple comes to experience how conjugal communion is enriched with those values of tenderness and affection which constitute the inner soul of human sexuality, in its physical dimension also. In this way sexuality is respected and promoted in its truly and fully human dimension, and is never 'used' as an 'object' that, by breaking the personal unity of soul and body, strikes at God's creation itself at the level of the deepest interaction of nature and person (par. 32).

In the second quotation are found some of the moral and pastoral concepts associated with the preaching and practice of the Church's teaching:

Married people too are called upon to progress unceasingly in their moral life, with the support of a sincere and active desire to gain ever better knowledge of the values enshrined in and fostered by the law of God. They must also be supported by an upright and generous willingness to embody these values in their concrete decisions. They cannot however look on the law as merely an ideal to be achieved in the future: they must consider it as a command of Christ the Lord to overcome difficulties with constancy. 'And so what is known as "the law of gradualness" or step-by-step advance cannot be identified with "gradualness of the law", as if there were different degrees or forms of precept in God's law for different individuals and situations. In God's plan, all husbands and wives are called in marriage to holiness, and this lofty vocation is fulfilled to the extent that the human person is able to respond to God's command with serene confidence in God's grace and in his or her own will. On the same lines, it is part of the Church's pedagogy that husbands and wives should first of all recognise clearly the teaching of *Humanae Vitae* as indicating the norm for the exercise of their sexuality, and they should endeavour to establish the conditions necessary for observing that norm. . . . It must also be kept in mind that conjugal intimacy involves the wills of two persons, who are however called to harmonise their mentality and behaviour: this requires much patience, understanding and time. Uniquely important in this field is unity of moral and pastoral judgment by priests, a unity that must be carefully sought and ensured, in order that the faithful may not have to suffer anxiety of conscience (par. 34).

Natural Family Planning

In the Church today the focus of interest is on those methods which have come to be referred to as Natural Family Planning (NFP). These methods which bring together a balance of unitive intercourse and periodic continence, focus the attention of man and woman together on their own fertility, which they jointly hold, in a manner which can lead to and maintain the experience of mutuality and personal sharing in their love making, and which heightens for them their awareness of spiritual and personal elements in the relationship. These methods can open a couple to the full physical and spiritual significance of their intimacy, described by Pope John Paul II at Limerick in these words: 'Respect the God-given cycle of life, for this respect is part of our respect for God himself, who created male and female, who created them in his own image, reflecting his own life-giving love in the patterns of their sexual being.'[18]

There would seem to be considerable reserve in the medical profession today concerning NFP. Hopefully, the studies being done worldwide will bring about a change of attitude. For the most part these studies are investigating the 'use effectiveness' of NFP, that is, their reliability as a method of fertility control in given populations. Some results have been encouraging, and some disappointing, although in all of them the basic 'method effectiveness' is being confirmed. This points to the need for more study in the emotional and motivational areas of sexual relationships, and NFP is particularly suited to an exploration of this *terra incognita* between men and women. There is, however, a small minority of couples for whom NFP is not suitable at the present time, notwithstanding motivation. This is a medical and a factual matter, and is no threat to the concept of NFP. In NFP most couples have to hand a most reliable method of family planning, given adequate motivation and instruction.

Sterilisation

The magisterium of the Church is clearly opposed to all direct sterilisation. The principal statement on this is the reply of the Congregation for the Doctrine of the Faith to the Bishops of the United States, *Sterilisation in*

Catholic Hospitals. This repeats the traditional position in the strongest terms:

> Therefore notwithstanding any subjectively right intention of those whose actions are prompted by the care or prevention of physical or mental illness which is foreseen or feared as a result of pregnancy, such sterilisation remains absolutely forbidden according to the Doctrine of the Church.[19]

Indirect sterilisation however is lawful and permitted by the Church, as is widely known. This term refers to an operation or procedure which is done to treat a pathological condition, and from which sterilisation follows as a necessary but not directly intended consequence. Examples of this include the removal of the womb if it is of itself a threat to health, or radiation treatment of the reproductive organs in the male or female for the treatment of associated cancer. We have seen this principle already as it applies to the indirect taking of life. There is one difference of opinion among traditional authors on this question and that concerns the removal of a scarred uterus which in the judgment of the doctor is now hazardous but not immediately threatening and certainly not capable, in his judgment, of bearing another child. The more conservative and majority view regarded hysterectomy in these circumstances as direct sterilisation, the contrasting and minority opinion regarded this operation as indirect and permissible.[20]

Exceptional Cases

It is the strictness or absoluteness of the Church's position on prevention of pregnancy that has been the focus of most of the questioning within the Catholic community. People have been concerned with what would seem to be the 'exceptional' cases of conscience, arising from serious pathology, or from genetic indications, or from difficult or impossible marital circumstances. In 1968 the Irish bishops wrote:

> We ask our people to believe that we are deeply and painfully aware of the delicate and personal problems and intellectual difficulties to which this teaching may give rise for some and we are especially conscious of the difficult decisions which may face doctors in particular cases. We ask that every effort should be made, by study and prayer, to appreciate and live the whole Catholic teaching on marriage and the family, and to see the condemnation of contraception in this life-giving context.[21]

There has been more than a decade of comment and reflection since *Humanae Vitae* and many of the difficulties which were expressed during those years are beginning to resolve themselves in the direction in which the Encyclical pointed. There are still, however, the 'difficult decisions' and the 'particular cases'. The most pressing of these cases today would be that of the couple who judge that they are gravely obliged in conscience not to conceive.

How might a grave obligation not to conceive arise? We have all probably heard of cases of people who have been warned not to become pregnant, and who have had a baby and survived. Perhaps the presence of such cases, and the reality of alarmist and dishonest diagnoses, have prevented us from giving adequate consideration to these issues. An obligation not to conceive could arise in the case of a woman who has been told, on the basis of a reasonable and honest diagnosis, that it would be a grave danger to her health to become pregnant. She might have serious heart disease or kidney disease. At the present time the Church will approve only of natural methods of fertility management, and there are some instances where these are not suited to particular couples.

As we have seen, the declaration *Sterilisation in Catholic Hospitals* takes a strict line in principle on this issue. It may be useful, however, to recall another aspect of Church teaching, namely the traditional recognition in moral theology of the judgment of the individual conscience in circumstances which are perplexing and which give a person grounds to believe that he or she may choose an exceptional course of action. At the time of the encyclical several hierarchies mentioned this teaching, and while the explicit context of their remarks refers, or may be supposed to refer, to contraception as such, in sufficiently grave circumstances their meaning could be taken to extend beyond this.

In their statement on the encyclical the Belgian bishops included this advice:

> Finally in dealing with the concrete application of certain directives of the moral order, it can happen that because of particular circumstances which appear to them as conflicts of duties some of the faithful sincerely believe that it is impossible for them to conform to these directives. In this case the Church asks them to seek loyally the mode of acting which will permit them to adapt their conduct to the given norms. If they do not succeed at first, they should not consider that because of this they are separated from God's love.[22]

The bishops of Canada said:

> Counsellors may meet others who, accepting the teaching of the Holy Father, find that because of particular circumstances they are involved in what seems to them a clear conflict of duties, e.g. the reconciling of conjugal love and responsible parenthood with the education of children already born or with the health of the mother. In accord with the accepted principles of moral theology, if these persons have tried sincerely but without success to pursue a line of conduct in keeping with the given directives, they may be safely assured that whoever

honestly chooses that course which seems right to him does so in good conscience.[23]

In their most recent statement on this matter the Irish bishops add the important precision 'freely chosen sexual intercourse' to their definition of the wrongness of contraception.[24] The statement of the Holy See *Sterilisation in Catholic Hospitals* makes the same point.[25] There are two distinct, but closely related aspects to this. The first of these is the reference to the traditional grounds in moral theology of diminished responsibility, namely force, fear and undue pressure. Secondly, and most importantly, where intercourse is not freely chosen, whether in marriage or outside of it, then contraception as such is not a violation of the marriage act, because 'the act' is itself gravely defective by virtue of the absence of mutual consent. In this kind of situation it is not contraception which is the moral problem; this resides rather in the state of mind of the husband or the offending male person.

Despite these various statements, it is difficult to get out of our minds the sense of defensiveness and frustration that can be engendered by controversy. I would like to conclude this section with a quotation from a recent article of my own in which I try to put a perspective on what has been happening:

> It is important to emphasise today how cognisant the Ordinary Magisterium has shown itself to be regarding the pastoral difficulties encountered in family planning. Both sides of the present divide tend to overlook this. There is a school of thought which is characterised by an impression that there are no problems at all, and that it is disloyal to suggest that there are. Even *Humanae Vitae* gives this the lie. On the other hand those who are offended by the mode in which the difficulties are acknowledged, and who resent the suggestion of weakness, sometimes fail to realise the exceptional extent to which the Magisterium has gone to reassure those who are experiencing difficulty that they are within the fold. When one stands back from the precise words and the nuanced language, the observer cannot but be struck by a very obvious conclusion: the encyclical and the Magisterium acknowledge the presence of a moral problem which is affecting the lives of many people, and they do so in a manner that is at pains not to cause any sense of exclusion whether from the practice of the faith or the sacramental means of grace. This is clearly the stated position. That it has not as clearly been the perceived position is a tragedy which has divided Catholics of every rank. *Humanae Vitae* pleaded not only for obedience, but for agreement, tolerance and charity.[26]

Conclusion

Looking back over what has been written, I am conscious not only of particular strands of argumentation and of questioning, but of a certain sensitivity to institutional changes and needs at the present time. It is not possible for any of us to stand outside of our moment in history. We are not martians, but creatures of Earth: doctors, teachers and clergy who are interacting with and relating to the demands and tensions of our own society, and the perceptions of those who have taught us and who have entrusted us with what we know. Perhaps the moral theologian is more conscious of this because his work is done in reference to a closely defined historical community within society, the Church.

When people read moral theology they expect to come into contact with the Church's teaching, and not only that, but they expect to get an understanding of this teaching. These are perfectly natural expectations. A close reading of a subject, however, brings to light not only some of the answers, but also, the full significance of some of the questions. There may be a new awareness of any obscurities or obstructions which lie in the way of full understanding.

I am reminded of the old maritime charts, which are still used, which include little drawings of the coastline as it appears from the sea. These drawings give a perspective on the approach to harbour which the map does not reveal. The good navigator will want the whole picture.

Changes within society, and within particular institutions, generate a momentum which is never completely subject to the control of one person. This momentum causes feelings of challenge, but also feelings of anxiety and of fear. These are sentiments which do not balance equally in different souls. Reproductive medicine touches upon a point of Christian sensitivity, and the unchristian and destructive attitudes which are present today make some good people blind to all the values of the age. When this happens, even the intelligent and concerned question is in danger of becoming a badge of disloyalty.

When Jesus answered questions he frequently met the questioner at a deeper level than that of the question. Time and time again he showed that he was coming at the whole thing from a more comprehensive viewpoint. The contribution that the moral theologian makes is sometimes of this order. He sets the individual conscience on the right track: he makes sure that the questions are the right questions, the starting points are the right starting points, the human priorities are the right human priorities. Jesus seemed always to be confident that once the issue was stated in its correct terms, then the questioner could arrive at the answer himself. This was the technique which he used on many occasions.

In this chapter I have attempted to do some of these things. However, if I may refer again to the good navigator, more than general directions are needed if the ship is to make port. Some directions must be precise and definite. There are times when one has to say 'This is wrong; you can't go that way.' This too is part of the Church's task, and the theologian's duty. It is part of the fabric of this chapter.

Finally, I refer to the individual judgment of conscience. Even when principles are clear their application calls for wise judgment. This is where experience comes in, bringing a quality that no book can describe. It is as true of medical judgments as it is of moral ones: skilled diagnosis alerts the doctor to what is really going on, as opposed to what appears to be the case. Moral judgment pins down the real issue in a particular situation and indicates what ought to be done.

Together, morals and medicine, in theory and in practice, focus on the best possible care of parents and of child.

Appendices

1

A Note on the Nursing Care of Congenitally Malformed Infants

JOSEPHINE MULLIGAN

Given that not every infant who suffers from severe congenital malformation is chosen for active management, then two distinct groups emerge in a specialised unit. These are:

1. A group receiving maximum treatment.
2. A group receiving palliative treatment, most of whom progress to terminal care.

During the past eight years I have been responsible for devising a nursing care programme for a unit which contains the above mentioned two groups of infants. I have observed that the co-existence of two such groups gives rise to many difficulties. These are:

i. strain and conflict within the health care team, bearing particularly on the nurse because of her pivotal position relative to the infants, the parents and the physicians;

ii. difficulty in deciding which are ordinary and extraordinary means of preserving life relative to each infant;

iii. helping parents to accept their deformed child and become involved in its nursing care;

iv. educating nurses and parents to the different aims of nursing care as practiced in group 1 and group 2. These aims are based on a distinction which is made between care of the acutely ill and care of the dying.

When a decision is made in favour of conservative management, as in group 2, all concerned must be committed to this – and they must be convinced that they are acting with integrity.

The ordinary requirements of each infant in this group must be met, and problems and discomforts which are specific to each stage of the infant's illness must be identified and relieved.

Parents should be encouraged to contribute to the comfort and care of the infant; a proper opportunity for bonding ought not to be hindered either by congenital malformation or by the demands of institutionalised nursing care.

If at any stage it becomes apparent that a change to active management would be in the medical interest of the child, this change is undertaken without hesitation.

Active surgical intervention is not precluded if such will add to the comfort of the child – e.g. the insertion of a shunt if hydrocephalus develops in an infant with spina bifida.

The nursing care of this infant includes:

1. Full caloric feeding, adjusting the amount and frequency to the infant's tolerance and condition. As the infant becomes weaker, adequate feeding may be continued by using a teaspoon or pipette. From my experience tube feeding is undesirable as it deprives the infant of an important source of pleasure, namely sucking, and it involves the discomfort of passing a tube on a regular basis.
2. Daily dressing of the open lesion.
3. Relief of any source of discomfort, with all the nursing expertise available.
4. Relief of pain and distress by the use of drugs in normal pharmacological doses, related to infant's weight.
5. Comfort which is afforded by personal contact and communication by parents and nurses with the infant.

As death approaches, the needs of both infant and family receive constant consideration; the personal involvement of the parents in affectionate caring is encouraged and supported right to the end.

2
Sacred Congregation for the Doctrine of the Faith: Declaration on Euthanasia

Introduction

The rights and values pertaining to the human person occupy an important place among the questions discussed today. In this regard, the Second Vatican Ecumenical Council solemnly reaffirmed the lofty dignity of the human person, and in a special way his or her right to life. The Council therefore condemned crimes against life 'such as any type of murder, genocide, abortion, euthanasia, or wilful suicide' (Pastoral Constitution *Gaudium et Spes*, 27).

More recently, the Sacred Congregation for the Doctrine of the Faith has reminded all the faithful of Catholic teaching on procured abortion.[1] The Congregation now considers it opportune to set forth the Church's teaching on euthanasia.

It is indeed true that, in this sphere of teaching, the recent Popes have explained the principles, and these retain their full force;[2] but the progress of medical science in recent years has brought to the fore new aspects of the question of euthanasia, and these aspects call for further elucidation on the ethical level.

In modern society, in which even the fundamental values of human life are often called into question, cultural change exercises an influence upon the way of looking at suffering and death; moreover, medicine has increased its capacity to cure and to prolong life in particular circumstances, which sometimes give rise to moral problems. Thus people living in this situation experience no little anxiety about the meaning of advanced old age and death. They also begin to wonder whether they have the right to obtain for themselves or their fellowmen an 'easy death', which would shorten suffering and which seems to them more in harmony with human dignity.

A number of Episcopal Conferences have raised questions on this subject with the Sacred Congregation for the Doctrine of the Faith. The Congregation, having sought the opinion of experts on the various aspects of euthanasia, now wishes to respond to the Bishops' questions with the present Declaration, in order to help them to give correct teaching to the faithful entrusted to their care, and to offer them elements for reflection that they can present to the civil authorities with regard to this very serious matter.

The considerations set forth in the present document concern in the first place all those whc place their faith and hope in Christ, who, through his life, death and Resurrection, has given a new meaning to existence and especially to the death of the Christian, as Saint Paul says: 'If we live, we live to the Lord, and if we die, we die to the Lord' (*Rom.* 14:8; cf. *Phil.* 1: 20).

As for those who profess other religions, many will agree with us that faith in God the Creator, Provider and Lord of life – if they share this belief – confers a lofty dignity upon every human person and guarantees respect for him or her.

It is hoped that this Declaration will meet with the approval of many people of good will, who, philosophical or ideological differences notwithstanding, have nevertheless a lively awareness of the rights of the human person. These rights have often in fact been proclaimed in recent years through declarations issued by International Congresses;[3] and since it is a question here of fundamental rights inherent in every human person, it is obviously wrong to have recourse to arguments from political pluralism or religious freedom in order to deny the universal value of those rights.

I. *The Value of Human Life*

Human life is the basis of all goods, and is the necessary source and condition of every human activity and of all society. Most people regard life as something sacred and hold that no one may dispose of it at will, but believers see in life something greater, namely a gift of God's love, which they are called upon to preserve and make fruitful. And it is this latter consideration that gives rise to the following consequences:

1. No one can make an attempt on the life of an innocent person without opposing God's love for that person, without violating a fundamental right, and therefore without committing a crime of the utmost gravity.[4]
2. Everyone has the duty to lead his or her life in accordance with God's plan. That life is entrusted to the individual as a good that must bear fruit already here on earth, but that finds its full perfection only in eternal life.
3. Intentionally causing one's own death, or suicide, is therefore equally as wrong as murder; such an action on the part of a person is to be considered as a rejection of God's sovereignty and loving plan. Furthermore, suicide is also often a refusal of love for self, the denial of the natural instinct to live, a flight from the duties of justice and charity owed to one's neighbour, to various communities or to the whole of society – although, as is generally recognised, at times there are psychological factors present that can diminish responsibility or even completely remove it.

   However, one must clearly distinguish suicide from that sacrifice of one's life whereby for a higher cause, such as God's glory, the salvation of souls or the service of one's brethren, a person offers his or her own life or puts it in danger (cf. *Jn* 15:14).

II. *Euthanasia*

In order that the question of euthanasia can be properly dealt with, it is first necessary to define the words used.

Etymologically speaking, in ancient times *euthanasia* meant an *easy death* without severe suffering. Today one no longer thinks of this original meaning of the word, but rather of some intervention of medicine whereby the sufferings of sickness or of the final agony are reduced sometimes also with the danger of suppressing life prematurely. Ultimately, the word *euthanasia* is used in a more particular sense to mean 'mercy killing', for the purpose of putting an end to extreme suffering, or saving abnormal babies, the mentally ill or the incurably sick from the prolongation, perhaps for many years, of a miserable life, which could impose too heavy a burden on their families or on society.

It is therefore necessary to state clearly in what sense the word is used in the present document.

By euthanasia is understood an action or an omission which of itself or by intention causes death, in order that all suffering may in this way be eliminated. Euthanasia's terms of reference, therefore, are to be found in the intention of the will and in the methods used.

It is necessary to state firmly once more that nothing and no one can in any way permit the killing of an innocent human being, whether a foetus or an embryo, an infant or an adult, an old person, or one suffering from an incurable disease, or a person who is dying. Furthermore, no one is permitted to ask for this act of killing, either for himself or herself or for another person entrusted to his or her care, nor can he or she consent to it, either explicitly or implicitly. Nor can any authority legitimately recommend or permit such an action. For it is a question of the violation of the divine law, an offence against the dignity of the human person, a crime against life, and an attack on humanity.

It may happen that, by reason of prolonged and barely tolerable pain, for deeply personal or other reasons, people may be led to believe that they can legitimately ask for death or obtain it for others. Although in these cases the guilt of the individual may be reduced or completely absent, nevertheless the error of judgment into which the conscience falls, perhaps in good faith, does not change the nature of this act of killing, which will always be in itself something to be rejected. The pleas of gravely ill people who sometimes ask for death are not to be understood as implying a true desire for euthanasia; in fact it is almost always a case of an anguished plea for help and love. What a sick person needs, besides medical care, is love, the human and supernatural warmth with which the sick person can and ought to be surrounded by all those close to him or her, parents and children, doctors and nurses.

III. *The Meaning of Suffering for Christians and the use of Painkillers*

Death does not always come in dramatic circumstances after barely tolerable sufferings. Nor do we have to think only of extreme cases. Numerous testimonies which confirm one another lead one to the conclusion that nature itself has made provision to render more bearable at the moment of death separations that would be terribly painful to a person in full health. Hence it is that a prolonged illness, advanced old age, or a state of loneliness or neglect can bring about psychological conditions that facilitate the acceptance of death.

Nevertheless the fact remains that death, often preceded or accompanied by severe and prolonged suffering, is something which naturally causes people anguish.

Physical suffering is certainly an unavoidable element of the human condition; on the biological level, it constitutes a warning of which no one denies the usefulness; but, since it affects the human psychological makeup, it often exceeds its own biological usefulness and so can become so severe as to cause the desire to remove it at any cost.

According to Christian teaching, however, suffering, especially suffering during the last moments of life, has a special place in God's saving plan; it is in fact a sharing in Christ's Passion and a union with the redeeming sacrifice which he offered in obedience to the Father's will. Therefore one must not be surprised if some Christians prefer to moderate their use of painkillers, in order to accept voluntarily at least a part of their sufferings and thus associate themselves in a conscious way with the sufferings of Christ crucified (cf. *Mt* 27:34). Nevertheless it would be imprudent to impose a heroic way of acting as a general rule. On the contrary, human and Christian prudence suggest for the majority of sick people the use of medicines capable of alleviating or suppressing pain, even though these may cause as a secondary effect semiconsciousness and reduced lucidity. As for those who are not in a state to express themselves, one can reasonably presume that they wish to take these painkillers, and have them administered according to the doctor's advice.

But the intensive use of painkillers is not without difficulties, because the phenomenon of habituation generally makes it necessary to increase their dosage in order to maintain their efficacy. At this point it is fitting to recall a declaration by Pius XII, which retains its full force; in answer to a group of doctors who had put the question: 'Is the suppression of pain and consciousness by the use of narcotics . . . permitted by religion and morality to the doctor and the patient (even at the approach of death and if one foresees that the use of narcotics will shorten life)', the Pope said: 'If no other means exist, and if, in the given circumstances, this does not prevent the carrying out of other religious and moral duties: Yes'.[5] In this case, of course, death is in no way intended or sought, even if the risk of it is reasonably taken; the intention is simply to relieve pain effectively, using for this purpose painkillers available to medicine.

However, painkillers that cause unconsciousness need special consideration. For a person not only has to be able to satisfy his or her moral duties and family obligations; he or she also has to prepare himself or herself with full consciousness for meeting Christ. Thus Pius XII warns: 'It is not right to deprive the dying person of consciousness without a serious reason.'[6]

IV. *Due Proportion in the use of Remedies*

Today it is very important to protect, at the moment of death, both the dignity of the human person and the Christian concept of life, against a technological attitude that threatens to become an abuse. Thus, some people speak of a 'right to die', which is an expression that does not mean the right to procure death either by one's own hand or by means of someone else, as one pleases, but rather the right to die peacefully with human and Christian dignity. From this point of view, the use of therapeutic means can sometimes pose problems.

In numerous cases, the complexity of the situation can be such as to cause doubts about the way ethical principles should be applied. In the final analysis, it pertains to the conscience either of the sick person, or of those qualified to speak in the sick person's name, or of the doctors, to decide, in the light of moral obligations and of the various aspects of the case.

Everyone has the duty to care for his or her own health or to seek such care from others. Those whose task it is to care for the sick must do so conscientiously and administer the remedies that seem necessary or useful.

However, is it necessary in all circumstances to have recourse to all possible remedies?

In the past, moralists replied that one is never obliged to use 'extraordinary' means. This reply, which as a principle still holds good, is perhaps less clear today, by reason of the imprecision of the term and the rapid progress made in the treatment of sickness. Thus some people prefer to speak of 'proportionate' and 'disproportionate' means. In any case, it will be possible to make a correct judgment as to the means by studying the type of treatment to be used, its degree of complexity or risk, its cost and the possibilities of using it, and comparing these elements with the result that can be expected, taking into account the state of the sick person and his or her physical and moral resources.

In order to facilitate the application of these general principles, the following clarifications can be added:

– If there are no other sufficient remedies, it is permitted, with the patient's consent, to have recourse to the means provided by the most advanced medical techniques, even if these means are still at the experimental stage and are not without a certain risk. By accepting them, the patient can even show generosity in the service of humanity.

– It is also permitted, with the patient's consent, to interrupt these means, where the results fall short of expectations. But for such a decision to be made, account will have to be taken of the reasonable wishes of the patient and the patient's family, as also of the advice of the doctors who are specially competent in the matter. The latter may in particular judge that the investment in instruments and personnel is disproportionate to the results foreseen; they may also judge that the techniques applied impose on the patient strain or suffering out of proportion with the benefits which he or she may gain from such techniques.

– It is also permissible to make do with the normal means that medicine can offer. Therefore one cannot impose on anyone the obligation to have recourse to a technique which is already in use but which carries a risk or is burdensome. Such a refusal is not the equivalent of suicide; on the contrary, it should be considered as an acceptance of the human condition, or a wish to avoid the application of a medical procedure disproportionate to the results that can be expected, or a desire not to impose excessive expense on the family or the community.

– When inevitable death is imminent in spite of the means used, it is permitted in conscience to take the decision to refuse forms of treatment that would only secure a precarious and burdensome prolongation of life, so long as the normal care due to the sick person in similar cases is not interrupted. In such circumstances the doctor has no reason to reproach himself with failing to help the person in danger.

Conclusion

The norms contained in the present Declaration are inspired by a profound desire to serve people in accordance with the plan of the Creator. Life is a gift of God, and on the other hand death is unavoidable; it is necessary therefore that we, without in any way hastening the hour of death, should be able to accept it with full responsibility and dignity. It is true that death marks the end of our earthly existence, but at the same time it opens the door to immortal life. Therefore all must prepare themselves for this event in the light of human values, and Christians even more so in the light of faith.

As for those who work in the medical profession, they ought to neglect no means of making all their skill available to the sick and the dying; but they should also remember how much more necessary it is to provide them with the comfort of boundless kindness and heartfelt charity. Such service to people is also service to Christ the Lord, who said. 'As you did it to one of the least of these my brethren, you did it to me' (*Mt* 25:40).

At the audience granted to the undersigned Prefect, His Holiness Pope John Paul II approved this Declaration, adopted at the ordinary meeting of the Sacred Congregation for the Doctrine of the Faith, and ordered its publication.

Rome, the Sacred Congregation for the Doctrine of the Faith, 5 May 1980.

Franjo Card. Šeper. *Prefect*

✠ Jérôme Hamer, O.P.,
Tit. Archbishop of Lorium, Secretary

3

Archdiocese of Dublin: Ethical Code for Hospitals

Preamble

1. This Ethical Code for Hospitals presents general guidelines for resolving some ethical issues which arise in hospitals at this time. It contains statements of general principle; it is not designed to provide a ready answer to every individual case. The concrete application of the principles to the particular case is a matter for the prudent judgment of conscience, which will take account of all the ethical factors in the situation.
2. This Code recommends that an ethical committee be established in each hospital in order to set out more clearly ethical policy, both for the day-to-day running of the hospital and for the problem cases.
3. The ethical principles in this Code necessarily take a summary and condensed form. Fuller and more detailed discussion of these principles and their applications may be found in the works of recognised authorities in the field of medical ethics.
4. Some of the ethical terminology in this Code is technical and may not be familiar to the non-specialist in ethics. It was, however, decided that accuracy of formulation was the primary concern.
5. This Code deals only with *some* of the ethical issues which arise in hospitals. The practice of medicine in hospitals inevitably touches on many other issues; their omission from this Code should not lead to the conclusion that they are considered unimportant.
6. While this Code finds its origin and inspiration in the Judaeo-Christian ethic, it is hoped that it will be acceptable not only to those who inherit that tradition but to all who deisre to maintain and promote genuine human values and standards in our society today.
7. Finally, this Code is a code for this time; it is not a code for all time. The progress of medical science constantly opens up new problems, so that more precise formulation of ethical principles may become both possible and necessary.

A. *The Hospital*

1. The hospital is an important focal point of moral responsibility and

ethical concern. It ought to offer a courageous witness to the highest ethical and moral principles. In the Christian tradition the hospital is committed to carrying on Christ's saving work, not only in healing and caring for the sick and injured but also in the positive promotion of good physical and mental health.

2. The concern of the hospital for the good of the patient is not confined to his bodily and mental welfare but extends to the spiritual wellbeing which is inseparably connected with bodily and mental welfare. Chaplains or other ministers should be appointed to provide for the spiritual wellbeing of the patients and should therefore have the support and co-operation of all in the hospital in the carrying out of an effective spiritual ministry.
3. Appropriate information, particularly concerning the dying, should be made available to those, of whatever denomination, responsible for the spiritual care of patients. Reasonable facilities for administering religious and sacramental care, to individuals or groups, should be provided, including the making available in the hospital of a suitable place for public worship.
4. No person can, in any circumstances, demand the use of hospital facilities for any operation, procedure, treatment or research which the hospital authority judges to be inconsistent with the ethical policy and accepted practices of the hospital.
5. Those who accept appointments or employment in any hospital should do so only on the understanding that they will not violate the ethical policy and accepted practices of the hospital.

B. *Principles of General Policy*

1. Every human being has the duty and right to preserve and maintain his life, physical and mental health and spiritual integrity. In the Christian view, these duties and rights are derived from God, the Creator, before whom man is the steward and custodian, not the absolute owner, of his life and destiny. From these basic duties and rights derive the responsibilities of all engaged in medical care, who must therefore respect each patient.
2. Medical intervention always requires the consent, at least implied or reasonably presumed, of the patient or his guardian. A patient ought always to be adequately informed of his condition; the responsibility to inform him rests primarily upon the doctor.
3. Medical intervention is justified in reference to medical or pathological need. A procedure producing damage or other negative effects in the patient is permitted when it is sincerely judged to be a necessary and proportionate means of remedying or containing a diseased condition.
4. The obligation of professional secrecy covers not only information on a patient's chart and records (howsoever preserved) but also confidential

matters learned in the course of professional duty.

5. No person may, in any circumstances, be required to participate in any way in an operation, procedure, treatment or research to which he has a conscientious objection; nor may he suffer any disability or discrimination whatsoever by reason of such conscientious objection.
6. Formal or willing co-operation in an immoral procedure is itself immoral. Material or unwilling co-operation may sometimes be justified by a proportionate reason.
7. To make for greater mutual understanding and co-operation among medical and nursing staff and to give guidance on problem cases, each hospital should have an ethical committee. It will be for the hospital authority to choose the members of this committee and to define its terms of reference. The ethical committee shall report to the hospital Board.

C. *Life and Death*

1. The moral task of the hospital is dominated by respect for human life and for the dignity of the human person. Respect for life cannot be separated from a special respect for the process of transmitting life which, in the Christian view, involves human persons in God's creative activity.
2. The human person, at every stage of life, is entitled to the protection of morality and law. Since life is particularly vulnerable in its beginning and ending, it is essential that the moments of conception and of death be as closely defined as medical science will allow and that these definitions be consistently adhered to.
3. Euthanasia, that is, the directly intended termination of a patient's life, even at his own request, is always morally wrong. The administration of sedatives or analgesics for the purpose of alleviating pain may be permitted for a proportionate reason, even if loss of consciousness or some shortening of life may result. Patients are to be supported and assisted in their dying and retain their rights to personal care until the moment of death has passed.
4. Failure to provide ordinary or reasonable means of preserving life is equivalent to euthanasia; but there is no obligation to use extraordinary or unreasonable means to prolong life.
5. Direct abortion, that is, any procedure the direct purpose of which is to prevent the implantation of the embryo or to remove it from the womb before it is viable, is immoral.
6. Operations and treatment necessary for the cure of serious organic pathological conditions of the mother, which cannot be postponed until the foetus is viable, are permitted even though the death of the foetus results. This principle applies also to extrauterine pregnancies.

D. *Other Issues*

1. The use of experimental surgical, medical or pharmacological procedures raises special moral issues. The hospital authority has overall responsibility for the ethical conduct of such procedures. All experimental procedures, including those carried out solely for purposes of research, require the informed and free consent of the patient.
2. In cases of organic transplant, the anticipated benefit to the recipient and the best interests of the donor must be fully considered. Vital organs may not be removed until death has taken place, the determination of the moment of death being made in accordance with the standard scientific criteria. As a safeguard in transplantation procedures, especially where the donor is unconscious, the team of doctors with responsibility for the recipient should be distinct from that responsible for the donor.
3. Procedures the direct purpose of which is to correct or prevent a seriously diseased organic condition are permitted even though they induce sterility.
4. Artificial insemination, that is, the attempt to bring about human conception outside of the marital relationship, is immoral. Appropriate medical assistance to enable parents to conceive is acceptable.

11th December 1978

4

Ethical Principles of the Coombe Lying-In Hospital, Dublin

Introduction. To make for greater mutual understanding and co-operation, and to give guidance on problem cases, the Board of Guardians and Directors has decided to appoint an Ethics Committee. The Committee is subject to the Board in every respect, and it shall be guided by the policy and traditions of the Coombe Hospital as set out here by the same Board.

The Policy and traditions which are here set out are statements of general principle which were drawn up following consultation with the medical and nursing staff; they are not designed to provide a ready answer to every individual case. The concrete application of principles to the particular case is a matter for the prudent judgment of conscience, which will take account of all the ethical factors in the situation.

1. *Consent:* Medical intervention always requires the consent, at least implied or reasonably presumed, of the patient or her guardian. A patient ought always to be adequately informed of her condition; the responsibility to inform her rests primarily upon the doctor.

2. *Mother and Baby:* The best interests of both mother and child is always to be considered, each being the subject of equal rights, whether before or after birth.

3. *Pathological Indication:* Medical intervention is justified in reference to medical or pathological need. A procedure producing damage or other negative effects in the patient is permitted when it is sincerely judged to be a necessary and proportionate means of remedying or containing a diseased condition.

   Procedures the direct purpose of which is to correct or prevent a seriously diseased organic condition are permitted even though they induce sterility.

Where there is a serious pathological contra-indication to pregnancy, a request for sterilisation, that is the directly intended inducement of sterility by surgical procedure, it is to be referred to the Master, who will have regard to policy as decided by the Board. This operation is excluded as a method of family planning.

4. *Secrecy:* The obligation of professional secrecy covers not only information on a patient's chart and records (howsoever preserved) but also confidential matters learned in the course of professional duty.
5. *Conscience:* No person may, in any circumstances, be required to participate in any way in an operation, procedure, treatment or research to which he/she has a conscientious objection; nor may he/she suffer any disability or discrimination whatsoever by reason of such conscientious objection.
6. *Beginning and end of life:* The human person, at every stage of life, is entitled to the protection of morality and law. Since life is particularly vulnerable in its beginning and ending, it is essential that the moments of conception and of death be as closely defined as medical science will allow and that these definitions be consistently adhered to.
7. *Life in the womb:* Direct abortion, that is, any procedure the direct purpose of which is to prevent the implantation of the embryo or to remove it from the womb before it is viable, is we believe immoral.

   Operations and treatment necessary for the cure of serious organic pathological conditions of the mother, which cannot be postponed until the foetus is viable, are permitted even though the death of the foetus results. This principle applies also to extrauterine pregnancies.
8. *Ordinary and extraordinary means of preserving life:* Euthanasia, that is, the directly intended termination of patient's life, even at the patient's own request, is always, we believe, morally wrong. The administration of sedatives or analgesics for the purpose of alleviating pain may be permitted for a proportionate reason, even if loss of consciousness or some shortening of life may result. Patients are to be supported and assisted in their dying and retain their rights to personal care until the moment of death has passed. Failure to provide ordinary or reasonable means of preserving life is equivalent to euthanasia; but there is no obligation to use extraordinary or unreasonable means to prolong life.
9. *Research:* The use of experimental surgical, medical or pharmacological procedures raises special moral issues. The hospital authority has overall responsibility for the ethical conduct of such procedures. All experimental procedures, including those carried out solely for purposes of research, require the informed and free consent of the patient.
10. *Assisting conception:* Artificial insemination with donor, that is, the attempt to bring about human conception outside of marriage, is, we

believe, immoral. Appropriate medical assistance to enable spouses to conceive is acceptable.

11. *Family planning:* We are committed to the education of patients in the knowledge and practice of family planning. We recognise that it is the couple rather than the individual who bear responsibility for family planning and we would, therefore, seek to serve the best interests of our patients in this regard. We further recognise that although reasonable provision will be made for patients in their choice of method, those methods which rely on the knowledge and use of natural cycles of fertility and infertility are most desirable from the point of view of good medicine, good health and personal well-being. Any method which is deemed to have, or deemed likely to have, an abortifacient effect, is excluded.

5

Excerpt from the Ethics Code of the Irish Medical Council

(COMHAIRLE NA nDOCHTUIRI LEIGHIS)

Constitution and Functions: A guide to ethical conduct and behaviour and to fitness to practise. (1981)

Reproductive Medicine. In an age of changing social, economic, political and philosophical attitudes the implications of scientific discoveries in the field of reproductive medicine present many new problems.

It is important for doctors to keep abreast of these developments which may have an important bearing on many aspects of patient care. These include – family planning, infertility, sterilisation, artificial insemination and the prevention of congenital handicap. In this whole area of conflicting attitudes, doctors while obeying the laws of the State, must always be guided by their own informed consciences.

Abortion in any circumstances is professional misconduct and it is illegal in the Republic of Ireland. Doctors must be prepared to resist requests by patients and their relatives to advise termination where pregnancy is unwanted.

There is evidence that a growing number of Irish women seek abortion from medical services outside the State. There is, thus, a special need for the profession to adopt a sympathetic and supportive role in caring for women presenting with unwanted pregnancies or pregnant women with disabling physical or psychological problems or where there is reason to believe that their baby will suffer from a congenital anomaly. The profession should encourage services for the support and care of mother and child. Doctors must maintain the time-honoured medical principle that every effort should be made to preserve human life, both born and unborn.

(pp.14–15)

Notes

Notes to Chapter 1, pp. 4–11

1. N.I.C.H.D. National Registry for Amniocentesis Study Group, 'Mid-Trimester Amniocentesis for Prenatal Diagnosis Safety and Accuracy', *J.A.M.A.*, 296 (1976) 1471–6.
2. See Working Party on Amniocentesis, 'An Assessment of the Hazards of Amniocentesis', *Brit. J. Obstet. Gynaecol.* 85/2 (1978); also M.P. Lamb, 'Gangrene of a Fetal Limb due to Amniocentesis', *Brit. J. Obstet. Gynaecol.* 82 (1975), 829–30; and also P.E. Young, M.R. Matson, O.W. Jones, 'Fetal Exsanguinations and Other Vascular Injuries from Mid-Trimester Genetic Amniocentesis', *Am. J. Obstet. Gynaecol.* (1977) 129–31.
3. See note 1, above.
4. See Working Party on Amniocentesis, note 2 above.
5. E.B. Hook and G.M. Chambers, 'Estimated Rates of Down's Syndrome in Live Births by One Year Maternal Age Intervals for Mothers aged 20–49' in *New York State Study Birth Defects*, 13/3A (1977), 124–41.
6. *Becher* v *Schwartz*, (1979) 47L W 2426.
7. Albert B. Gerbie, Seminar in Perinatology, vol. IV, no. 3, 1980.
8. See note 7, above.
9. J.A. Murken, *Proceedings of 3rd European Conference on Pre-natal Diagnosis of Genetic Disorders*, Stuttgart 1979.
10. R.M. Fineman *et al.*, *Nature*, 260 (1976), 320–21; also P.J. Fialkow, 'Thyroid Antibodies; Down's Syndrome and Maternal Age', *Nature*, 214, (1967), 1253–4.
11. S.A. Rhine *et al.*, 'A Simple Alternative to Amniocentesis for First Trimester Prenatal Diagnosis', *Birth Defects*, 12/31 (1977), 231–47.
12. J. Schroeder, 'Transplacental Passage of Blood Cells', *J. Med. Genet.*, 12 (1975), 230–42.

Notes to Chapter 2, pp. 12–20

1. C.O. Carter, 'Genetic Counselling', *Brit. J. Hosp. Med.* (1978), 557–62.
2. Seymour Kessler, ed., *Genetic Counselling: Psychological Dimensions*, Dublin: Academic Press, 1979.
3. J.H. Tjio and A. Levan, 'The Chromosome Number of Man', *Hereditas* (Lund), 42 (1956), I.
4. P.S. Harper, *Practical Genetic Counselling*, Bristol: Wright, 1st ed. 1981, 93–4.

Notes to Chapter 3, pp. 21–31

1. U.S. Dept of Health and Human Services Study, Centre for Disease Control, *Abortion Surveillance 1978*, (1980).
2. J.J. Rovinsky and S.B. Gusberg, *Am. J. Obstet. Gynaecol.*, 98 (1967), 11.
3. M.K. O'Driscoll, C.F.V. Coyle and M.I. Drury, *Br. Med. J.*, II (1962), 767.
4. J. Bonnar, *Pregnancy Hypertension*, London: M.T.P. Press, 1980.
5. N. Walsh, *Studies* (1972), 303.
6. Hook, *Acta Psychiat. Scandinav.* 39, Supp. 168 (1963).
7. J.A. Stallworthy, A.S. Moolgaoker and J.J. Walshe, *Lancet*, II (1971), 1245; see also S.M. Karim and A. Filshie, *J. Obstet. Gynaecol. Br. Commonw.*, 79 (1972), 1; M.P. Embrey, K. Hillier and P. Mahendron, *Br. Med. J.*, III (1972), 146; and J.E. Hodgson, R. Smith and D. Milstein, *J. Amer. Med. Ass.*, 228 (1974), 849.
8. The Church Assembly Board for Social Responsibility, *Abortion – An Ethical Discussion*, 1965, 61.

Notes to Chapter 5, pp. 45–52

1. D.M. de Kretser, *Clinics in Obstetrics and Gynaecology*, I (1974), 409.
2. Pius XII, address: 'Vegliare con Sollectudine', to the Italian Association of Catholic Midwives, 1951.
3. J. Mahoney, S.J., in *The Month* (October 1978), 329.
4. P.C. Steptoe, R.G. Edwards and J.M. Purdy, *Br. J. Obstet. Gynaecol.*, 87 (1980), 757.
5. B. Haring, *Ethics of Manipulation*, 1975, 192.

Notes to Chapter 7, pp. 74–86

1. Dorothy Scally, 'Natural Family Planning – The Hidden Agenda', *CMAC Bulletin*, 80/20 (October 1980), 5–11.

Notes to Chapter 9, pp. 95–117

1. [1974] I.R. 284 (Sup. Ct., 1973). For analysis of the decision, see Dooley, *Soc. Studies*, 3 (1974), 186; O'Reilly, *Studies*, 65 (1977); Binchy, *Studies*, 65 (1977), 330.
2. *Griswold* v *Connecticut* (1965) 381 U.S. 479.
3. *Eisenstadt* v *Baird* (1972) 405 U.S. 438.
4. Dittfurth, 'Judicial Reasoning and Social Change' (1975) 50 Indiana L.J. 258, at 273.
5. Abortion Act 1967.
6. *Roe* v *Wade* (1973) 410 U.S. 113; see also *Doe* v *Bolton* (1973) 410 U.S. 179.
7. Judgment of 25 February 1975, (1975) 39 BVerfG 1–95. See Kommers, 'Abortion and Constitution: United States and West Germany', 25 Am. J. Comp. L 255 (1977); Gorby, Jonas and Kommers, 'West German Abortion Decision: A Contrast to Roe v

Wade'; J. Marshall in (1976) 9 J. of Practice and Procedure 551; Destro, 'Abortion and the Constitution: The Need for a Life Protective Amendment' (1975) 63 Calif. L. Rev. 1250.

8. First sentence of article II(2) of the Basic Law.
9. In German: 'Jeder hat das Recht auf Leben'.
10. Supra, n.7. It should be noted that the Court's judgment did not involve a finding that abortion would be illegal in all circumstances. Since the judgment, different legislation providing for abortion in certain cases has been enacted: see Horton, 'West German Abortion Reform – One Year Later' (1978) 8 Family L. 62.
11. The Court in its Judgment referred specifically to this background.
12. See Veitch, 'Delicta in Uterum' (1972) 24 N.I.L.O. 40; Winfield, 'The Unborn Child' (1942) 8 Camb. L.J. 76; Gordon, 'The Unborn Plaintiff', (1965) 63 Mich. L. Reg. 579; Samuels, 'Comment: Injuries to Unborn Children' (1974) 12 Alta. L. Rev. 266; Mathews, 'Quantitative Interference with the Right to Life: Abortion and Irish law' (1976) 22 Catholic L. 344; Pace, 'Civil Liability for Pre-Natal Injuries' (1977) 40 Modern L. Rev. 141.
13. Cf. *Walker* v *G.N. Ry.*, 28 L.R. Ir. 69 (Q.B.).
14. Offences Against the Person Act 1861, section 58 (24 and 25 Vict., c.100). Procuring or supplying drugs or an instrument with intent to cause an abortion is also an offence: ibid., section 59. See further Russell on *Crime*, vol. 1, 602–5 (12th ed., by J. Turner, 1964).
15. [1939] 1 K.B. 687, analysed by Seaborne Davis, 'The Law of Abortion and Necessity' (1939) 2 Modern L. Rev. 126; see also B. Dickens, *Abortion and the Law*, 1966, 38ff.; M. Simms and K. Hindell, *Abortion Law Reformed*, 1971, 13–14, 69–72; R. Cook and B. Dickens, *Abortion Laws in Commonwealth Countries*, 1979, 8–9, 13ff.; G. Williams, *Textbook of Criminal Law*, 1978, 254–5.
16. E.G. Veitch and Treacy, 'Abortion in the Common Law World' (1974) 22 Amer. J. Comp. L., 652, at 654; Exshaw, 'Some Illustrations of the Application and Meaning of "Unlawful" in Criminal Law' [1959] Crim. L. Rev. 503, at 507–08; Maksymiuk, 'The Abortion Law: A Study of *R.* v *Morgentaler*' (1975) 39 Sask. L. Rev. 259, at 265; Quay, 'Justifiable Abortion – Medical and Legal Foundations' (1961) 49 Georgetown L.J. 395, at 435.
17. Most notably Professor Glanville Williams of Cambridge: see G. Williams, *The Sanctity of Life and the Criminal Law*, 1958, 151ff.; G. Williams, *Criminal Law: The General Part*, 2nd ed. 1961, 730–31.
18. Section 1(1) of the Act. For analyses of the Act and its origins, see K. Hindell and M. Simms, *Abortion Law Reformed*, 1971; Hart, 'Abortion Law Reform: The English Experience' (1972) 8 Melbourne U.L. Rev. 388.
19. Ibid., section 1(2).
20. This is apparent from the debates of the Standing Committee of the House of Commons on Mr John Corrie's Abortion (Amendment) Bill, November 1979 to February 1980.
21. (1973) 410 U.S. 113; see also *Doe* v *Bolton* (1973) 410 U.S. 179. The decision led to a flood of commentary. Helpful analyses include Byrn, Wade and Bolton, 'Fundamental Legal Errors and Dangerous

Implications' (1973) 19 Catholic L. 243; O'Meara, 'The Court Decides a Non-Case' [1973] Sup. Ct. Rev., 337; Goodman, Schoenbroad and Steavis, 'Doe and Roe: Where Do We Go From Here?' (1973) 1 Women's Rts. L. Reptr. 20; Ely, 'The Wages of Crying Wolf: A Comment on *Roe* v *Wade*' (1973) 82 *Yale L.J.* 920; Haley, 'Haunting Shadows From the Rubble of Roe's Right of Privacy' (1974) 9 Suffolk U.L. Rev. 145; Satris, 'Roe! Doe! Where are you? The Effect of the Supreme Court's Abortion Decisions' (1974) 7 U. Calif. Davis L. Rev. 432.

22. Cf. section 1(1) of the English Abortion Act 1967, which permits abortion where there is a substantial risk that if the child were born it would suffer from 'such physical or mental abnormalities as to be seriously handicapped'.
23. Drinan, 'The Inviolability of the Right to be Born', in *Abortion, Society and the Law*, ed. D. Walbert and J. Butler, 1973, 123, at 130.
24. Sergeant, infra, n.26, at 788, citing Marks and Salkovitz, 'The Defective Newborn: An Analytic Framework for a Policy Dialogue', in *Ethics of Newborn Intensive Care*, 1976, 110–11; see also Nobel Prize winner James Watson's statement that 'most birth defects are not discovered until birth. . . . [If] a child were not declared alive until three days after birth, all parents could be allowed the choice [to preserve the child's life] that only a few are given under the present system': Watson, 'Children from the Laboratory', *Prism* (May 1973) at 12–13; cf. Tooley, 'Abortion and Infancticide' (1972) 2 Phil. and Public Affairs 37, at 44, arguing that an 'organism possesses the concept of a self as a continuing subject of experiences and other mental states, and believes that it is itself such a continuing entity'. For more recent analyses of the moral and legal issues, see McCormick, 'Human Life and Human Rights', ch. 6 of *Understanding Human Rights: An Interdisciplinary and Interfaith Study*, ed. A. Falconer, 1980; Campbell and Duff, 'Deciding the Cases of Severely Malformed or Dying Infants', *J. Med. Ethics*, 5 (1979), 65; King, 'Defective Babies and Death by "Natural Causes"', *The Guardian*, 16 March 1981.
25. (1973) 410 U.S. 113
26. Sergeant, 'Withholding Treatment from Defective Newborns: Substituted Judgment, Informed Consent, and the Quinlan Decision' (1978) 13 Gonzaga L. Rev. 781.
27. McIntyre, 'Genetic Risk, Prenatal Diagnosis, and Selective Abortion', in *Abortion, Society and the Law*, ed. D. Walbert and J. Butler, 1973, 223, at 224.
28. Cf. Swan, 'Compulsory Abortion: Next Challenge to Liberated Women' (1975) 3 Ohio N.L. Rev. 152.
29. Supra, pp.100–101.
30. J.M. Kelly, *The Irish Constitution*, 1980, 374 (emphasis added).
31. O'Reilly, 'Marital Privacy and Family Law', *Studies* (Spring 1977), 8, at 17.
32. *McGee* v *A.G.* [1974] I.R. 284.
33. *G.* v *An Bord Uchtala*, 113 I.L.T.R. 25.
34. O'Reilly, 'Marital Privacy and Family Law', *Studies*, 65 (1977), 8, at 8.

35. Ibid., at 17.
36. Casey, 'The Development of Constitutional Law Under Chief Justice O Dalaigh' [1978] Dublin U.L.J. 1, at 10.
37. (1972) 405 U.S. 438.
38. Kelly, *Irish Constitution*, 343. An injunction was granted against the State in *Bohan* v *Garda Commissioner, A.G. Ireland*, unreported, *Irish Times*, 7 March 1981, 18.
39. Therapeutic sterilisation is beyond the scope of the present article.
40. This aspect of the law is discussed neither by Mr Alan Shatter in his recent text on family law, *Family Law in the Republic of Ireland* (1977) nor by Mr O'Siochain in the most recent edition of his text on criminal law, *Criminal Law of Ireland* (6th ed. 1977), for example.
41. Shartel and Plant, *The Law of Medical Practice*, 1959, 144, quoted in Wolf, 'Legal Psychiatric Aspects of Voluntary Sterilization' (1963) 3 J. Family L. 103, at 118.
42. Bravenec, 'Voluntary Sterilization as a Crime: Applicability of Assault and Battery and of Mayhem' (1966) 6 J. Family L. 94.
43. J. Smith and B. Hogan, *Criminal Law*, 2nd ed., 1969.
44. J. Smith and B. Hogan, supra, n.43, 253.
45. Cf. J. Smith and B. Hogan, supra, n.43; 255ff. Williams, 'Consent and Public Policy' [1962] Crim. L. Rev. 74, 154; Hughes, 'Two Views on Consent in the Criminal Law' (1963) 26 Modern L. Rev. 233.
46. J. Smith and B. Hogan, surpra, n.43, 255.
47. Ibid.
48. Cf. *R.* v *Coney* (1882) 8 Q.B.D. 534, at 539. Where a player is assaulted intentionally on the pitch, however, this may give rise to criminal and civil liability on the part of his assailant, as a recent successful prosecution in England has demonstrated.
49. [1954] 1 W.L.R. 1169.
50. Supra, n.48, at 549.
51. Supra, n.49, at 1176.
52. Supra, n.49. Denning L. J's view was strongly criticised by Hughes, supra, n.45, at 238–9 and Williams, supra, n.45, at 157.
53. See, e.g. D. Meyers, *The Human Body and the Law: A Medico-Legal Study*, 1970, 12–19; Skegg, 'Medical Procedures and the Crime of Battery', [1974] Crim. L. Rev. 694, at 694ff.
54. J. Smith and B. Hogan, supra, n.43, 257.
55. [1974] I.R. 294 (Sup. Ct., 1973).
56. Cf. *Jessin* v *County of Shasta*, 274 Cal. Appl 2d 737, 79 Ca. Reptr. 359 (Dist. Ct. App., 1969); Bloom, 'Comment: A Woman's Right to Voluntary Sterilization' (1972) 22 Buffalo L. Rev. 291, at 303; Forbes, 'Voluntary Sterlization of Women as a Right' (1969) 18 De Paul L. Rev. 560, at 564–5.
57. Referred to generally as artificial insemination homologous.
58. Referred to generally as artificial insemination heterologous.
59. See A. Shatter, *Family Law in the Republic of Ireland*, 1977, 63ff.
60. Ibid., 75, 159. See also *L.* v *L.* [1949] P.211, and J. Jackson, *The Formation and Annulment of Marriage*, 2nd ed. 1969, 348–50.
61. Cf. A. Shatter, supra, n.59, 63–4.
62. Cf. Holloway, 'Artificial Insemination: An Examination of the Legal

Aspects' (1957) 43 Am. Bar. Assoc. J. 1089, at 1090.

63. *Orford* v *Orford*, 49 Ont. L. R. 15, 58 D.L.R. (Sup. Ct., Orde, J., 1921), discussed by Tallin, 'Artificial Insemination', (1956) 34 Can. Bar Rev. 1, 166; Hubbard, id., 425, and Guttmacher, 'The Legitimacy of Artificial Insemination' (1946) 11 Human Fertility 16 at 17.
64. Maclenan v. Maclenan [1958] S.C. 105, analysed by Payne, 'Artificial Human Insemination', (1958) 12 N. Ireland L.Q. 252, at 260–61; Bartholemew, 'Legal Implications of Artificial Insemination' (1958) 21 Modern L. Rev. 236, at 251–2; E. Clive and J. Wilson, *The Law of Husband and Wife in Scotland*, 1974, 447–50; and Oakley, 'Test Tube Babies: Proposals for Legal Regulation of New Methods of Human Conception and Pre-Natal Development' (1974) 8 Family L.Q. 385, at 387. The decision provoked a debate in the House of Lords but (as yet) no legislative response in Britain.
65. Cf. ibid., at 109–10: 'In the normal and natural method of performing an act of sexual intercourse there is a mutual surrender both of the sexual and reproductive organs. While the primary purpose of sexual intercourse is procreation, in the eyes of the law surrender of the reproductive organs is not necessary to consummate the act of intercourse. Expedients may be used by the parties to secure birth prevention, or the woman may have previously undergone an operation by which her reproductive organs were removed, or they may have ceased to function from natural causes; and yet the conjunction of the sexual penetration would constitute intercourse and, in the circumstances under consideration, adultery. Thus impregnation *per se* cannot be a test of adultery, since in the eyes of the law the act of intercourse can be consummated without impregnation, either as a result of natural casues or by the parties resorting to artificial expedeints (cf. *Baxter* v *Baxter*, [1948] A.C. 274). It would seem therefore that, in determining such questions as consummation of marriage or adultery, the law looks at the act and not at the result.'
66. In *Doornbus* v *Doornbus* (1954) 23 U.S. Law Week 2308, app. dismissed 12 Ill. App. 2d 473, 139 N.E. 2d (1954); the Superior Court of Cook County, Illinois, held that adultery had been committed but in *Hoch* v *Hoch*, unreported, (1945), the opposite view had been taken by the same court: see Weinberger, 'A Partial Solution to Legitimacy Problems Arising From the Use of Artificial Insemination', (1960) 35 Indiana L. Rev. 143, at 146, Massey, 'Comment: Artificial Insemination: The Law's Illegitimate Child?' (1963) Villanova L. Rev. 77, at 78; H. Krause, *Illegitimacy and Social Policy*, 1971, 18–19.
67. See, e.g., Weinberger, supra, n.57, at 147, who criticises *Orford* v *Orford*, supra, n.63, for being 'completely at variance with the well-recognised commom law definition [of adultery]'.
68. *Orford* v *Orford*, supra, n.63, at 22 and 258, respectively.
69. Cf. Van Einden, 'Comment: Artificial Insemination and the Problem of Legitimation and Adultery' (1955) U. Illinois L. Forum 759, at 761.
70. See generally Shatter, *Family Law in the Republic of Ireland*, 117ff.
71. Dienes, 'Artificial Donor Insemination: Perspectives on Legal and

Social Change' (1968) 54 Iowa L. Rev. 253, at 265.

72. See Report of the Departmental Committee on Human Artificial Insemination, paras. 160–71 (1960) Cmnd. 1105; Mayo, 'Legitimacy for the A.I.D. Child' (1974) 6 Family Law 19; C. Pincher, *Sex in Our Time*, 1973, 178–9; Cusine, 'A.I.D. and the Law', I J. of Med. Ethics (1975) 39, at 39; Stone, 'English Law in Relation to A.I.D. and Embryo Transfer', in *CIBA Foundation Symposium, Law and Ethics of A.I.D. and Embryo Transfer* (1973), 69, at 71. In the United States, some decisions have held the child to be legitimate: see, e.g., *Strnad* v *Strnad*, (1948) 78 N.Y.S. 2d 390 (discussed by Holloway, supra, n.13, at 1091), but there have been holdings to the contrary: see e.g., *Gursky* v *Gursky*, 242 N.Y.S. 2d 406 (Sup. Ct., 1948), *Anon.* v *Anon.*, 246 N.Y.S. 835 (Sup. Ct., 1964), discussed by Smith, 'Through a Test Tube Darkly: Artificial Insemination and the Law' (1968) 67 Michigan L. Rev. 127, at 136–7.
73. For a discussion of the difficulties facing a person seeking to establish the illegitimacy of the child of his spouse, see A. Shatter, supra, n.59, 157–9.
74. Ibid., 335–7.
75. See the Family Law (Maintenance of Spouses and Children) Act 1976, Sections 3(1) and 5 (no. 11 of 1976).
76. Ibid., section 3(1); see further, Binchy, 'Family Law Reform in Ireland: Some Comparative Aspects' (1976), 25 International and Comparative L.Q. 901; cf. a somewhat similar development in California, accomplished by 'judicial legislation' in *People* v *Sorensen* (1968) 66 Cal. Rptr. 7, 437 P. 2d 495, analysed by Sherman, 'Note: *People* v *Sorensen:* Artificial Insemination Gives Birth to Real Problems in California', 4 Calif. W.L. Rev. 177.
77. Vital Statistics and Births, Deaths and Marriages Registration Act 1952, section 2(4), (no. 8).
78. Supra, n. 77.
79. Ibid., section 2(4).
80. Cf. the remarks of Lord Denning, *Parl. Debs. H.L.* (26 Feb. 1958), vol. 207, col. 945.
81. Cf. Kenny's *Outlines of Criminal Law*, 18th ed., by J. Turner, 1962, 421–2.
82. Halsbury's *Laws of England*, 4th ed., by Lord Hailsham of St Marylebone, 1976, vol. II, para. 61.
83. Cf. the Legitimacy Act 1931, section 9(1) (no. 13).
84. *Mens rea* may be difficult to establish. Cf. Halsbury, supra, n.76, para. 60. But see the remarks of Lord Denning, supra, n.80, cols. 944–6, and Goldfarb, 'Artificial Insemination: The Legal Viewpoint' (1955) 7 Syracuse L. Rev. 108, at 113.
85. This is the present law in Ireland since, before maintenance obligations towards a child can be imposed on a man who is not the father of the child, he must be aware of this fact.
86. *Parl. Debs.* vol. 207, col. 944.
87. Ibid., paras. 945–6.
88. Cf. Goldfarb, supra, n. 84, at 113; and Lord Denning, supra, n. 80, col. 946.

89. 'Report of Panel on Human Artificial Insemination', *Br. Med. J. Supplement*, vol. 2 (1973), 3, at 4.
90. Cf. A. Holder, *Medical Malpractice Law*, 2nd ed. 1978, 250.
91. See Pennington and Naik, 'Donor Insemination: Report of a Two-Year Study', *Br. Med. J.* vol. 1 (1977), 1327, at 1328.
92. See O. Stetler and A. Mortiz, *Doctor and Patient and the Law*, 4th ed., 1962, 104–5. Cf. Pennington and Naik, supra, n.91, at 1327, who canvass the possibility of the child's right of action where he is born with a defect; see also 'Report of Panel on Human Artificial Insemination', supra, n.89 at 4.
93. Of course, a customary practice, even where established, does not control: cf. *O'Donovan* v *Cork Co. Co.*, [1967], I.R. 173, at 193–4 (Sup. Ct., per Walsh, J., 1965).

Notes to Chapter 10, pp. 118–145

1. J. Fletcher, *Situation Ethics*, Philadelphia 1966, 133.
2. J. Lejeune, in *Ethical Issues in Human Genetics*, ed. Hilton et al., New York – London 1973, 113.
3. 'Report of the Committee set up by the Irish Medical Association to advise on the Modes of Action of Intrauterine Devices', *Journal of the Irish Medical Association*, vol. 73 no. 5 (May 1980), 188–90.
4. Pro-Life Amendment Campaign, Dublin, May 1981: the present Irish Government has stated its intention of holding a referendum on such an amendment, March 1982.
5. K. Lebacz, 'Pre-Natal Diagnosis and Selective Abortion', in *Linacre Quarterly*, 40 (1973), 109–27, and reprinted in *Ethics in Medicine*, ed. Reiser, Dyck, Curran; Cambridge (Mass.) 1977, 376–87, 384.
6. L. Kass, 'Implications of Pre-Natal Diagnosis for the Human Right to Life', in op. cit. *Ethical Issues in Human Genetics*, ed. Hilton *et al.*, 185–99, 178.
7. See 'Death, Definition and Determination of', in *Encyclopedia of Bioethics*, editor-in-chief W.T. Reich, New York 1978, 292–307.
8. The problem of selection is discussed in the book *Decision Making and the Defective Newborn. Proceedings of a Conference on Spina Bifida and Ethics*, ed. C.A. Swinyard, Springfield Illinois, 1978. Best known of the objective criteria are those proposed by J. Lorber, 'Results of the Treatment of Myelomeningocele'. *Developmental Medicine and Child Neurology*, 13 (1971), 279–303; id. 'Early Results of Selective Treatment of Spina Bifida Cystica', *British Medical Journal* 4 (October 27, 1973), 201–4; id. 'Selective Treatment of Myelomeningocele: To Treat or Not to Treat?', *Pediatrics*, 53 (March 1974), 307–8.
9. The concept of objective criteria has been challenged by R.M. Veatch, 'The Technical Criteria Fallacy', and by R. Reid, 'Spina Bifida: The Fate of the Untreated', in *The Hastings Center Report*, vol. 7, no. 4 (August 1977), 15–16 and 16–19. See also Appendix: Josephine Mulligan, 'A Note on The Nursing Care of Infants with Congenital Malformations not amenable to Surgical Intervention'.
10. W.T. Reich, in op. cit., *Decision Making and The Defective Newborn*, 489–511.

11. In a recent article 'Human Life and Human Rights' (in *Understanding Human Rights: An Interdisciplinary and Interfaith Study*, ed. Alan D. Falconer, Dublin 1980, 74–84) Richard A. McCormick S.J.. adds four 'specifying rules' to a criterion for decision-making in this area which he put forward in an earlier article ('To Save or Let Die', *Journal of the American Medical Association* 229/2, 8 July 1974, 172–6). The criterion originally proposed read: 'If that potential (for relationships) is simply non-existent or would be utterly submerged and undeveloped in the mere struggle to survive, that life has achieved its potential.' This led to considerable debate in the following years, and the specifying rules given now by Fr McCormick reduce greatly the grounds for controversy and add considerable precision to his initial proposal.
The four specifying rules are:
1. Life-saving interventions may not be omitted for institutional or managerial reasons. Included in this specification is the ability of *this particular family* to cope with a badly disabled baby. This is likely to be a controversial guideline because there are doubtless many who believe that the child is the ultimate victim when parents unsuited to the challenge of a disadvantaged baby must undertake the task, still, it remains an unacceptable erosion of our respect for life to make the gift of life once given depend on the personalities and emotional or financial capacities of the parents alone. No one may be allowed to die simply because *these parents* do not feel up to an arduous task. At this point society has some responsibilities.
2. Life-saving interventions may not be omitted simply because the baby is retarded. There may be further complications associated with retardation that justify withholding life-sustaining treatment. But retardation alone is not an indication.
3. Life-sustaining interventions may be omitted or withdrawn at some point when it becomes clear that expected life can be had only for a relatively brief time and only with continued use of artificial feeding forever.
4. Life-sustaining interventions may be omitted or withdrawn when there is excessive hardship, especially when this combines with poor prognosis (e.g. repeated cardiac surgery, low prognosis transplants).

12. See for example K. Rahner, 'Experiment with Man', *Theological Investigations*, New York 1972, vol. IX, 205–24, and ibid. 'The Problem of Genetic Manipulation', op. cit., 225–52. See discussion and criticisms of these in J.M. Gustafson, *The Contribution of Theology to Medical Ethics*, Marquette University Theology Department, 1975, 47–54.

13. P.E. McKeever, 'Artificial Insemination', in *New Catholic Encyclopedia*, New York 1967, vol. 1, 922–4.

14. Address to Fourth International Congress of Catholic Doctors, 29 Sept. 1949, A.A.S., 1949, XLI, 559; Address to the Congress of The Association of Catholic Midwives (Vegliare Con Sollecitudine), 29 Oct. 1951, A.A.S., 1951, XLIII, p. 850; Address to the Second World Congress on Fertility and Sterility, 19 May 1956, A.A.S., 1956, XLVIII, pp. 470–71.

15. For further statement of this argumentation see: J. Mahoney, 'Ethical Horizons of Human Biological Development', *The Month* (1978), 329–33, 331. For similar opinions see: B. Häring, *Medical Ethics*, London 1972, 93; M. Di Ianni, 'Fecondazione Artificiale', in *Dizionario Enciclopedico di Teologia Morale*, Rome 1974, 401–12, 409; this article contains an extensive bibliography of theological writing on this question; in the same volume, see L. Rossi, 'Masturbazione', 614–25, 617; M. Vodipivec, 'Samensuntersuchung', in *Lexikon für Theologie und Kirche*, Freiburg 1974, vol. IX, 296. Notice also the comment on The Declaration on Certain Questions concerning Sexual Ethics, which reaffirms traditional Catholic teaching on masturbation, without referring to this kind of case, by D. O'Callaghan, in *The Furrow*, vol. 27/2 (February 1976), 126–8.
16. *Gaudium et Spes*, 50; *Humanae Vitae*, 10; *Familiaris Consortio*, 28.
17. The Synod Propositions, 21, in *The Tablet*, 31 January 1981, 118; see *Familiaris Consortio*, 29.
18. *The Pope in Ireland*, Addresses and Homilies, Dublin 1978, 80.
19. Translation from *The Linacre Quarterly* (August 1976), 210–11.
20. For a discussion on these points see: T.J. O'Donnell, 'Sterilization', in *New Catholic Encyclopedia*, vol. 13, 704–5; K. Lebacz, 'Sterilization: Ethical Aspects', in *Encyclopedia of Bioethics*, 1609–1613; J.T. Noonan, *Contraception*, Harvard 1965, chapter XIV, 451–60; The minority view is held by J.C. Ford and G. Kelly, *Contemporary Moral Theology*, vol. II, New York 1963, 328–37.
21. Statement 9 October 1968, *Humanae Vitae and the Bishops*, ed. Horgan, Shannon (Ireland) 1972, 138–9.
22. Statement 30 August 1968, *Humanae Vitae and the Bishops*, op. cit., 66.
23. Statement 27 September 1968, *Humanae Vitae and the Bishops*, op. cit., 81.
24. Statement 16 October 1980, on The Health (Family Planning) Act 1979.
25. Par. 3 refers to 'sexual actions deliberately performed'.
26. M. Reidy, 'Moral Theology and Family Planning', *The Furrow*, vol. 32, no. 6, June 1981, 343–61, 347.

Notes to Appendix 2, pp. 151–157

1. *Declaration on Procured Abortion*, 18 Nov. 1974: *AAS* 66 (1974), 730–47.
2. Pius XII, *Address to those attending the Congress of the International Union of Catholic Women's Leagues*, 11 Sept. 1947: *AAS* 39 (1947), 483; *Address to the Italian Catholic Union of Midwives*, 29 Oct. 1951: *AAS* 43 (1951), 835–54; *Speech to the members of the International Office of military medicine documentation*, 19 Oct. 1953: *AAS* 45 (1953), 744–54; *Address to those taking part in the IXth Congress of the Italian Anaesthesiological Society*, 24 Feb. 1957: *AAS* 49 (1957), 146, cf. also *Address on 'reanimation'*, 24 Nov. 1957: *AAS* 49 (1957), 1027–33; Paul VI, *Address to the members of the United Nations Special Committee on Apartheid*, 22 May 1974: *AAS* 66 (1974),

346; John Paul II: *Address to the Bishops of the United States of America*, 5 Oct. 1979: *AAS* 71 (1979), 1225.

3. One thinks especially of Recommendation 779 (1976) on the rights of the sick and dying, of the Parliamentary Assembly of the Council of Europe at its XXVIIth Ordinary Session; cf. *SIPECA*, No. 1, March 1977, 14–15.
4. We leave aside completely the problems of the death penalty and of war, which involve specific considerations that do not concern the present subject.
5. Pius XII, *Address* of 24 Feb. 1957: *AAS* (1957), 147.
6. Pius XII, ibid., 145; cf. *Address* of 9 Sept. 1958: *AAS* (1958), 694.